Naert / van Steenberghe/Worthington, Osseointegration in Oral Rehabilitation

Osseointegration in Oral Rehabilitation
An Introductory Textbook

Edited by

Ignace Naert, D.D.S., Ph.D.
Associate Professor
Department of Prosthetic Dentistry
Faculty of Medicine
Catholic University Leuven
Leuven, Belgium

Daniel van Steenberghe, M.D., D.D.S., Ph.D.
Professor
Department of Periodontology
Faculty of Medicine
Catholic University Leuven
Leuven, Belgium

Philip Worthington, M.D., D.D.S.
Professor
University of Washington
School of Dentistry
Department of Oral and Maxillofacial Surgery
Seattle, Washington, U.S.A.

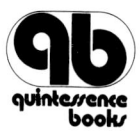

Quintessence Publishing Co., Ltd. 1993
London, Chicago, Berlin, São Paulo and Tokyo

British Library Cataloguing in Publication Data

Osseointegration in Oral Rehabilitation
I. Naert, Ignace Eugeen
617.6

ISBN 1-85097-030-0

Lithograpy: JUP Industrie- und Presseklischee, Berlin
Composition, Printing and Binding: Bosch-Druck, Landshut

Printed in West Germany

ISBN 1-85097-030-0

Contributors

P.G.F.C.M. Battistuzzi D.D.S., Ph.D.
Associate Professor
University of Njimegen
Philips van Leydenlaan 25
Postbus 9101
NL-6500 HB Njimegen, The Netherlands

P.-I. Brånemark,
M.D., Ph.D., Professor
Institute for Applied Biotechnology
Box 5411
S-402 29 Gothenburg, Sweden

J.B. Brunski, Ph.D., Associate Professor
Biomedical Engineering Department
Rensselaer Polytechnic Institute
Troy, New York 12180-3590, U.S.A.

G.E. Carlsson, Odont. Dr. Professor
Department of Prosthetic Dentistry
Faculty of Odontology
University of Gothenburg
Medicinaregatan 12,
S-413 90 Gothenburg, Sweden

L. Chen, D.M.D.
Universität Zürich
Zahnärztliches Institut
Abteilung für Kronen- und Brücken-
Prothetik, Teilprothetik und Materialkunde
Plattenstraße 11
CH-8028 Zürich, Switzerland

D. Harris, F.D.S., M.R.C.S., L.R.C.P.
School of Dental Science
Trinity College Dublin and
Centre for Tissue Integrated Reconstruction
The Blackrock Clinic
Blackrock, Dublin, Ireland

J.-E. Hausamen, Dr. Dr., Professor
Medizinische Hochschule Hannover
Klinik und Poliklinik für
Mund-, Kiefer- und Gesichtschirurgie
Postfach 61 01 80
D-3000 Hannover 61, Germany

S. Karlsson, Odont. Dr.
Associate Professor
Department of Prosthetic Dentistry
Faculty of Odontology
University of Gothenburg
Medicinaregatan 12,
S-413 90 Gothenburg, Sweden

B. Kasemo, Professor
Dept. of Applied Physics
Chalmer University of Technology
S-412 96 Gothenburg, Sweden

Th. Kerschbaum, Dr. Professor
Klinik und Poliklinik für Zahn-,
Mund- und Kieferheilkunde
der Universität zu Köln
Kerpener Straße 32
D-5000 Köln 51, Germany

J. Lausmaa, Professor
Dept. of Applied Physics
Chalmer University of Technology
S-412 96 Gothenburg, Sweden

I.E. Naert, D.D.S., Ph.D.,
Associate Professor,
Department of Prosthetic Dentistry
Faculty of Medicine
Catholic University Leuven
Kapucijnenvoer 7
B-3000 Leuven, Belgium

F.W. Neukam, P.D., Dr. Dr.
Medizinische Hochschule Hannover
Klinik und Poliklinik für
Mund-, Kiefer- und Gesichtschirurgie
Postfach 61 01 80
D-3000 Hannover 61, Germany

M. Quirynen, D.D.S., Ph.D.,
Associate Professor
Department of Periodontology
Faculty of Medicine
Catholic University Leuven
Kapucijnenvoer 7
B-3000 Leuven, Belgium

W.E. Roberts, D.D.S., Ph.D.,
Professor and Chairman
Indiana University
School of Dentistry
Department of Orthodontics
1121 West Michigan Street
Indianapolis, Indiana 46202-5186, U.S.A.

P. Schärer, D.M.D., M.S., Professor and
Chairman
Universität Zürich
Zahnärztliches Institut
Abteilung für Kronen- und Brücken-
Prothetik, Teilprothetik und Materialkunde
Plattenstraße 11
CH-8028 Zürich, Switzerland

H. Schliephake, Dr., Dr.
Medizinische Hochschule Hannover
Klinik und Poliklinik für
Mund-, Kiefer- und Gesichtschirurgie
Postfach 61 01 80
D-3000 Hannover 61, Germany

R. Skalak, Ph.D., Professor
Institute for
Biomedical Engineering
Room 5601, Engineering Building Unit
La Jolla, California 92093-0412, U.S.A.

J.-F. Tulasne, M.D., Dr.
26, Avenue Kléber
F-75116 Paris, France

D. van Steenberghe, M.D., D.D.S.,
Ph.D., Professor and Head of the
Department of Periodontology
Faculty of Medicine
Catholic University Leuven
Kapucijnenvoer 7
B-3000 Leuven, Belgium

Ph. Worthington, M.D., D.D.S., Professor
and Chairman
University of Washington
School of Dentistry
Department of Oral and Maxillofacial
Surgery
Seattle, Washington 98195, U.S.A.

Contents

Preface

The successful replacement of lost natural teeth by means of tissue-integrated implants represents a major advance in clinical treatment. Our knowledge and understanding of oral endoprostheses has evolved from the laboratory phase into clinical practice over the past three decades. It is essential that the dentists of the future are taught this subject at undergraduate level, since it will become an important aspect of clinical care. This will also ensure that they do not have to attend commercial courses after graduation without the necessary background knowledge.

This book aims to help dental students to integrate prosthetic rehabilitation, with or without implant support, into their clinical practice. For this reason, the team approach is emphasized, and it is made clear that implants are only one of a number of possible solutions to a problem.

The contributors to the volume all agreed to participate with great enthusiasm, and we are greatly indebted to our colleagues for this ready commitment. These chapters were produced at the cost of precious time by people who already face too many demands, owing to their acknowledged scientific and teaching skills.

Chapter 1

Introduction

L. Chen and P. Schärer

What is osseointegration?

Osseointegration is defined as direct bone anchorage to an implant body, which will provide a foundation to support a prosthesis; it is able to transmit occlusal forces directly to the bone[1, 2, 3].

What does it mean for the patient?

It is possible to replace lost soft and hard tissue and to rehabilitate and improve chewing function and oral comfort. Even the best fitting full denture cannot offer the same stability, chewing comfort and increase in self-confidence as a fixed implant-supported prosthesis[4].

There are increasing numbers of people with dental problems, as life expectancy increases in our society. The standard of living has also increased over the last decades, so that many people are no longer willing to accept removable partial or full dentures.

Among young people, on the other hand, there has been a marked decrease in dental decay. Nevertheless, sporting accidents and congenitally missing teeth are quite frequent, and these patients also, demand tooth preserving procedures such as oral implants.

For these reasons, there is a constantly growing demand for implants. In the past few years many systems have been introduced onto the market. The practising dentist, unfortunately, has been forced to rely on promotional literature from the various manufacturers of implant systems, and here, commercial interests often obscure scientific facts.

Many patients have therefore been treated with implant systems based on few scientific facts and little long-term observation.

The lack of scientific background knowledge is a particular problem, because the loss of an implant may, in the worst cases, require rehabilitative surgery to rebuild the supporting tissues to their previous level.

For implant therapy to be successful, the factors which determine success or failure should first be evaluated: that is the "software" (patient, dentist) and the "hardware" (the implant system). Success seems to depend on these three factors. In untrained hands, even the best implant system can fail, although improvements in the materials over recent years have clearly reduced the clinical failure rate. A "triangle" can therefore be postulated.

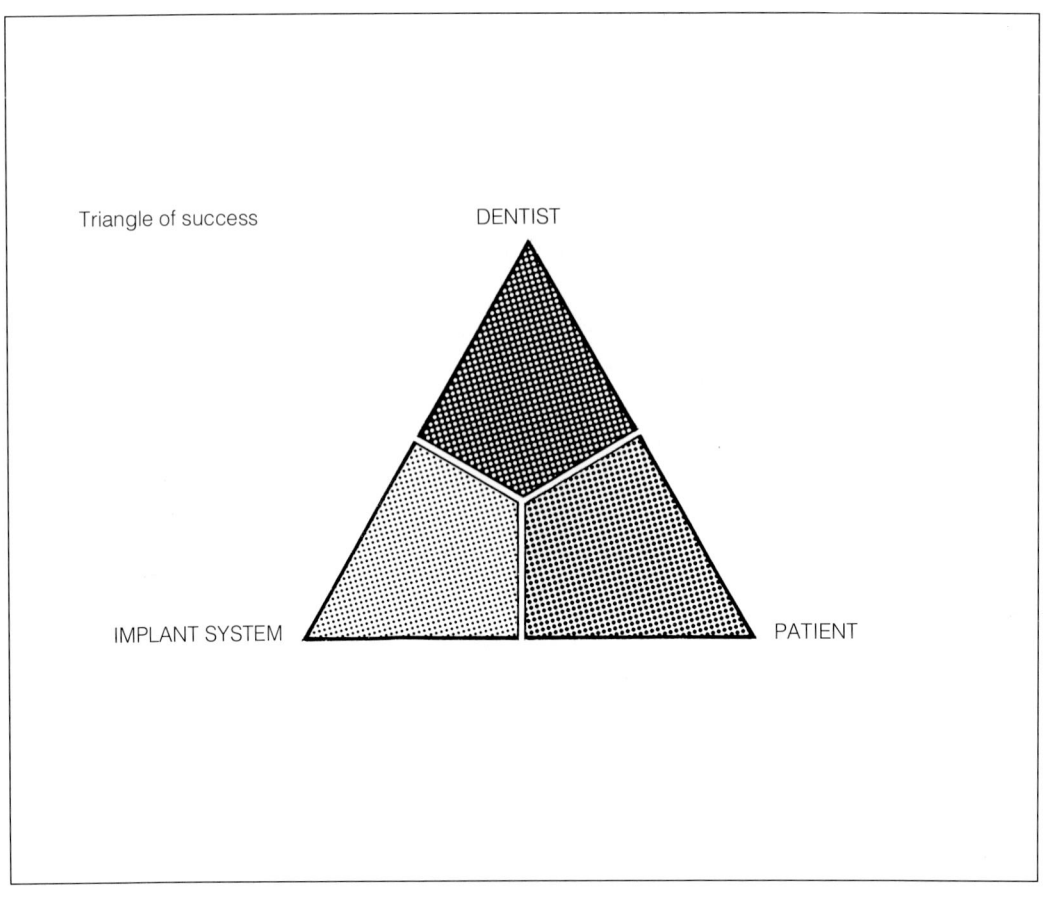

Triangle of success

DENTIST

IMPLANT SYSTEM

PATIENT

If any one part of the "triangle of success" is inadequate, the final outcome of the clinical procedure may be adversely affected.

A critical evaluation of each part of the "success triangle" will therefore be of interest.

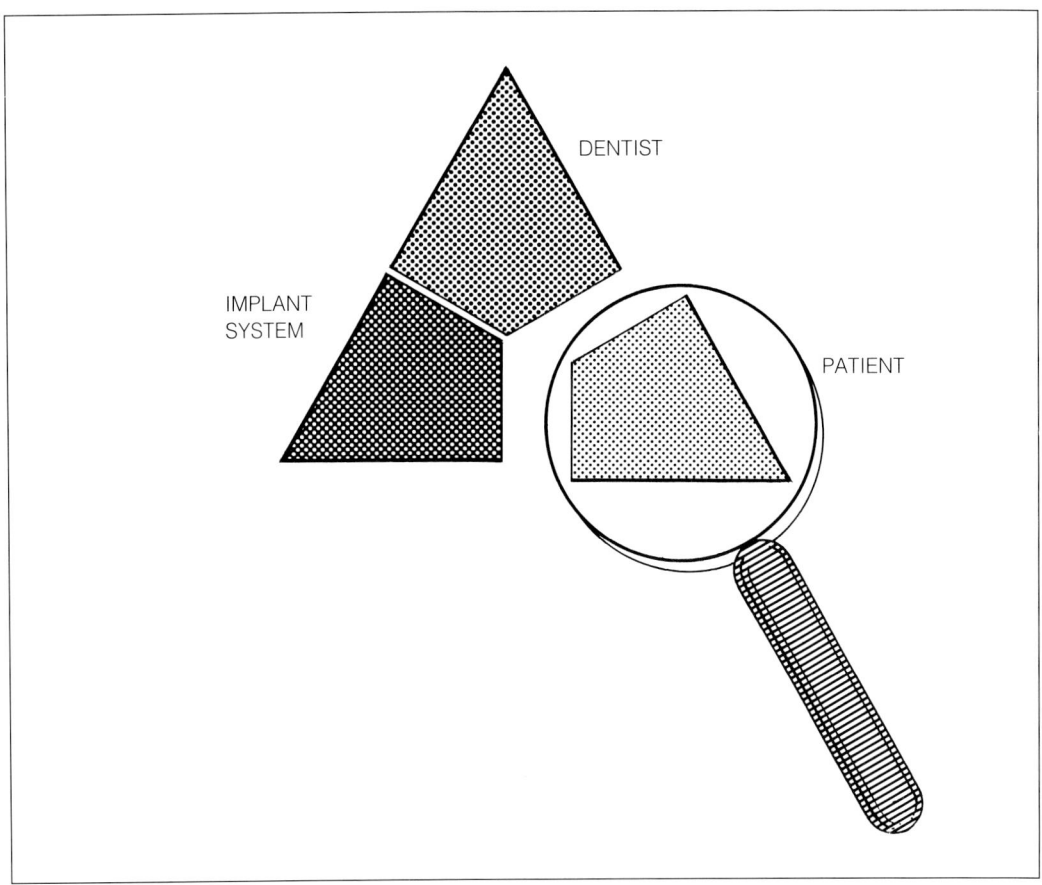

Patient

Indications

(1) Motivated, cooperative, good oral hygiene;
(2) Growth of alveolar process; completed (after the age of 16 years).

Contraindications

Absolute contraindications include:
(1) Severe systemic disorders;
(2) Psychiatric disease (e.g. psychoses, dysmorphobia);
(3) Alcoholics, drug abusers.

Relative contraindications include:
(1) Insufficient volume of bone for implant placement;
(2) Poor bone quality;
(3) Patients undergoing radiation treatment;
(4) Insulin-dependent diabetes;
(5) Heavy smokers.

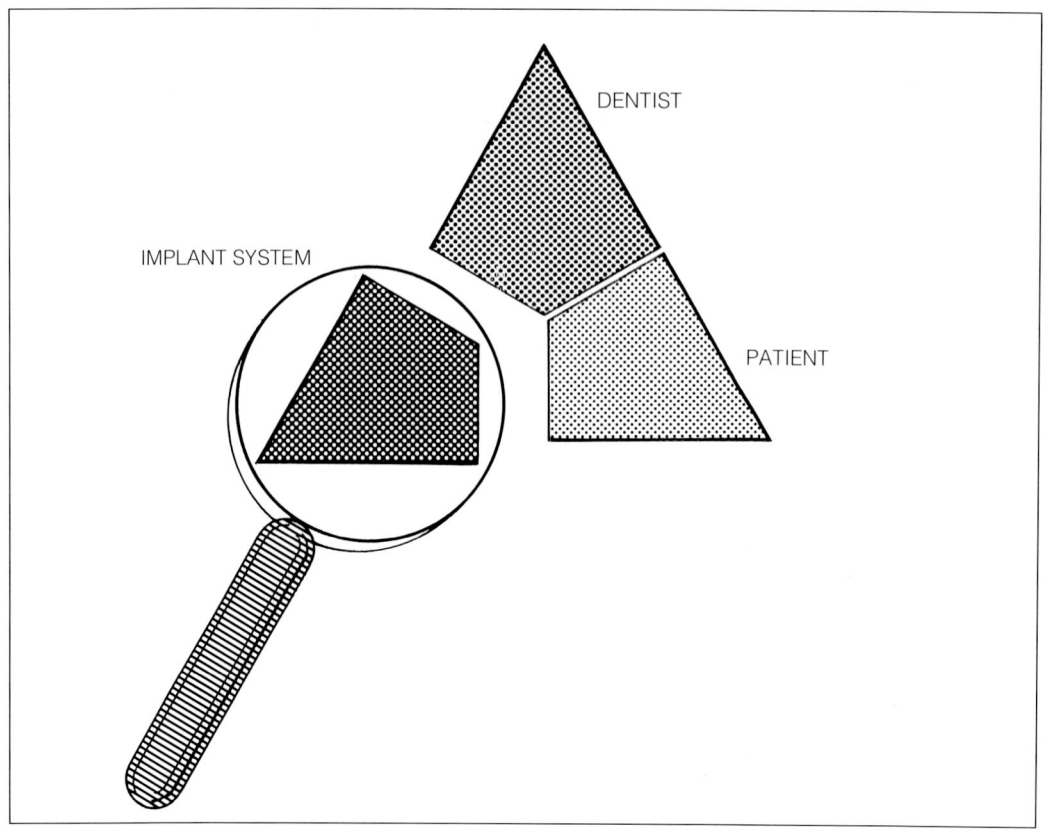

Implant system

Historical review

Attempts to replace lost teeth date back a long way: *Andrews* (1893) describes root-shaped obsidian implants made by Maya Indians (100–1500 AD). In the 19th century dentists experimented with different allo-plastic materials; *Maggiolo* (1809), *Hilli-scher* (1891), and *Zamensky* (1891) tried using gold, porcelain and India rubber. However, they were not very successful.

The first system reported to be satisfactory was constructed by *Greenfield*[5]. His patented iridioplatinum lattice implant was probably the first clinically applicable en-dosteal implant system.

Screw-type implants

Strock (1939) replaced single teeth with chrome cobalt screws. *Formiggini* (1947), and later *Chérchève* (1962), used double helical implants. All were constructed using metal (cobalt chrome, titanium, or stainless steel). *Linkow* (1963) introduced the Vent-Plant, a vented screw-type implant. The first ones were made of chrome cobalt, tantalum or stainless steel. In 1964, he began to make them using a titanium-based alloy.

In 1952, in the Vital Microscopy Laboratory at the University of Lund, Sweden, *Per-Ing-var Brånemark* and his team investigated blood rheology and wound healing, using titanium observation chambers. More or less by chance, they discovered the bio-compatible nature of titanium. After encouraging results with animal experiments, the first patients were treated with screw-shaped pure titanium implants in 1965.

In 1969, *Brånemark* et al.[6] described direct bone contact with a metallic implant, and in 1977[7] coined the term osseointegration for this phenomenon. The clinical criteria for successful osseointegration have been described by *Albrektsson* et al.[8]. Osseointegration on the ultrastructural level is still being investigated[9] (see chapter 5₁).

Cylindrical or root-shaped implant bodies

These were proposed by *Kirsch* and *Koch* (1977), *Schroeder* et al. (1976), and *Schulte* and *Heimke* (1976). They are made using aluminium oxide, plasma sprayed titanium and hydroxyapatite-coated titanium.

Blade-type implants

For patients with knife-edged, shallow or resorbed ridges, *Linkow* (1967) developed the Blade-Vent implant. This has a flat, blade-shaped and perforated design.

Subperiosteal implants

Earlier this century, *Müller* (1937), *Dahl* (1947), and *Gershkoff* (1949) developed subperiosteal implants. However, they produced very discouraging long-term results, with severe bone resorption following failure (*Bodine,* 1977, *Obwegeser,* 1977).

The basic criteria which should be fulfilled by each implant system are listed below.

The implant

Biocompatibility

The following biomaterials have been successfully tested for osseointegration:
Titanium[11]
Zirkonium[12]
Niobium
Hydroxyapatite[13]

Strength

Titanium and its alloys appear to be the material of choice. Ceramics are brittle and their use as oral implants may be limited to coatings. Stability of coatings is still being investigated[14].

Design

Tissue damage. There should be minimal bone and soft tissue damage following failure or removal of an implant; designs with extensions should be avoided.

Initial stability. Screw-type implants and slightly conical porous designs show good initial resistance to shear stress, this is a prerequisite for successful osseointegration[15].

Surface

Anchor effect. Implants with minor surface irregularities become better anchored to bone than otherwise identical smooth implants[16, 17].

Maintenance. In cases of peri-implant bone loss, macro- or micro-irregularities may become a problem.

Summary

The best implant system, according to the above criteria, involves the use of a biocompatible material and a screw-type design with minor surface irregularities (e.g. sandblasted/micro grooved).

Equipment

Drilling instrumentation

Standard instruments with burs of increasing diameter are necessary for the preparation of implant sites within bone; this can be carried out by hand or by machine.

The use of drilling instruments of progressively increasing diameter will minimize thermal injury to the osseous tissues[18, 19]. Disparities between the implant bed and the implant cannot be bridge the gap greater than 0.35–0.85 mm[20].

Cooling

A suitable internal or external cooling system, and sterile physiological saline solution should be used, to avoid thermal damage. Temperatures above 47 °C lead to necrosis and resorption of bone[21].

Packaging

Suitable packaging is necessary to ensure sterile delivery of the implants, and should specify the sterilization date and the period of ensured sterility.

Packaging which enables implantation to be carried out without undesirable contact with the implant surface, will help to avoid contamination[22].

Long-term studies

Albrektsson et al.[23] defined acceptable success rates (i.e. adequate retention time in function) as 85% at the end of a 5-year observation period and 80% at the end of a 10-year period.

Costs

For patients with a low income, basic equipment, implants and prosthetic parts should be available within a reasonable price range.

Prosthetics

Impression taking

The final restoration should fit without creating any tension on the abutments. Furthermore, the impression procedure must be as atraumatic as possible. In order to achieve these goals, well fitting transfer-copings and abutment replicas are needed, in order to provide a precise reproduction of the intra-oral conditions in the working model.

Precision fitting

An exact wax model of the prosthetic framework can best be developed on the abutments and abutment replicas; these should have a definite margin (e.g. shoulder).

Prosthetic versatility

A selection of prosthetic parts for
(a) a fixed prosthesis (single tooth, bridges), or (b) a removable prosthesis (overdentures, partial dentures) should be available.

Hygiene and maintenance

In order to facilitate hygiene, abutment length should be variable, in order to compensate for different soft tissue thicknesses. The diameter should permit a correct emergence profile, and the surface must be smooth.

Summary

A number of essential accessories are necessary for impression taking and the fabrication of superstructures with optimal precision fit and contours (hygiene).

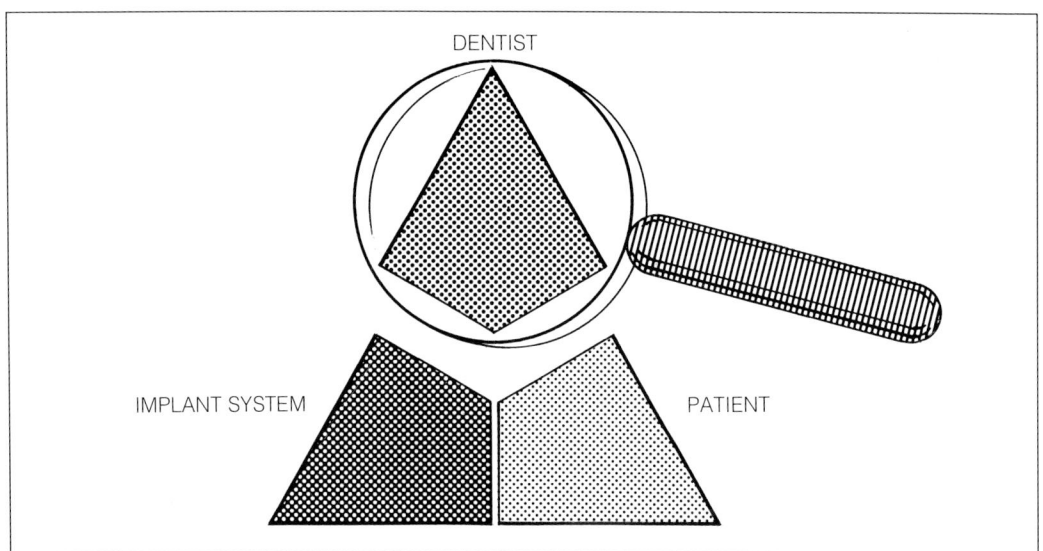

DENTIST

IMPLANT SYSTEM

PATIENT

The Dentist

Treatment planning

Rehabilitation by means of implants requires a multidisciplinary approach. The restorative goals must first be defined by the prosthodontist, and prosthetic alternatives evaluated. The surgeon must accept that implant placement depends not only on the bone and space available, but primarily on optimal prosthetic and occlusal conditions. Guides such as surgical stents can help the surgeon with site selection for implant placement.

Alternatives to implants

Single tooth replacement

Biological considerations. By using implants, restorative treatment may be limited to the edentulous space, with no involvement of neighbouring teeth required. The use of a fixed partial denture (FPD) requires the preparation of two teeth for one pontic area. If neighbouring teeth are already in need of restorative treatment, an FPD might be indicated.

17

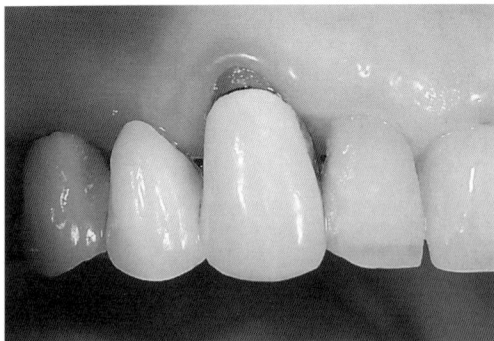

Fig. 1. Female patient (aged 73) on presentation. Failing FPD 13–15 owing to vertical root fracture of 13 with soft tissue break down.

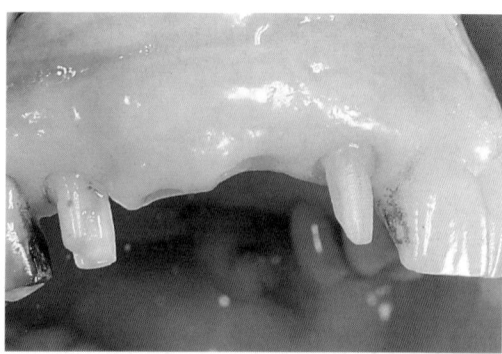

Fig. 2. Same patient after preparation of teeth 15, 12 and 11 for FPD and soft tissue grafting procedure. The 11 is prepared for a bonded metal wing.

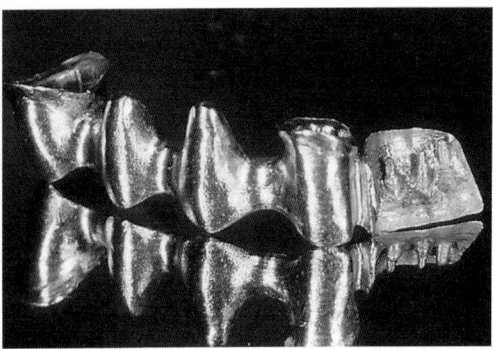

Fig. 3. Framework design for FPD. Because 11 is free of dental decay, it will support the bridge by means of a palatal bonded wing.

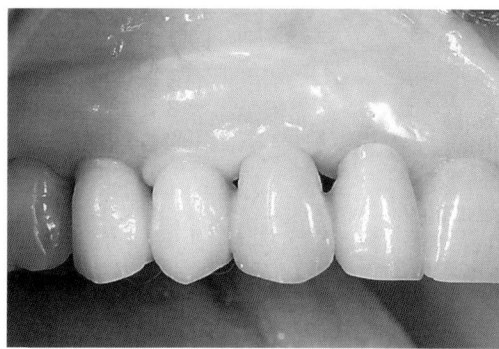

Fig. 4. The final result. Note the emergence profile of pontics 14 and 13. The illusion of a sulcus can be created by using ovate pontics.

Aesthetic considerations. Many patients will demand an aesthetically perfect result, wherever their smile line is located. Aesthetically, the use of an FPD to replace a single tooth gives excellent results. Using grafting procedures (e.g. subepithelial grafts, full-thickness grafts, roll flaps) and ovate pontics, the results can be optimized.

Using modern techniques such as Maryland bridges (adhesive retained bridges), even the loss of tooth substance through tooth preparation can be minimized.

The current high aesthetic standards seen in FPD replacements should be used as a baseline when planning for single tooth implants. In aesthetically important areas (e.g. upper anterior teeth in high lip-line patients) this requires careful diagnosis, particularly with regard to:
(1) Optimal bone relationship (6 mm x 6 mm x 10 mm);
(2) Soft tissue anatomy;
(3) Smile line.

Based on these diagnostic criteria, any pretreatment, such as site development (e.g.

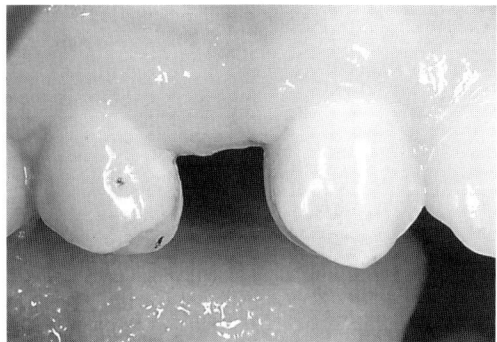

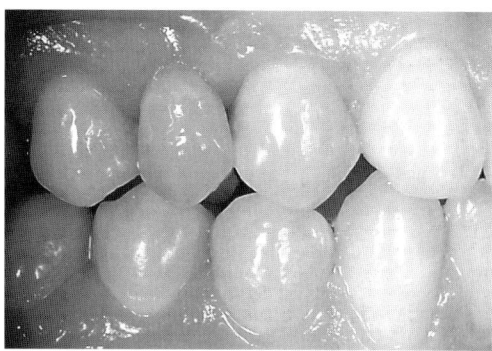

Fig. 5. Female patient (aged 18). The 13 lies in the position of the congenitally missing 12, with an edentulous space between 13 and 14.

Fig. 6. Result after insertion of a resin-bonded bridge at 14–13.

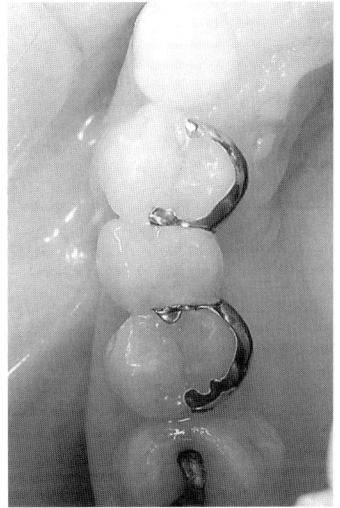

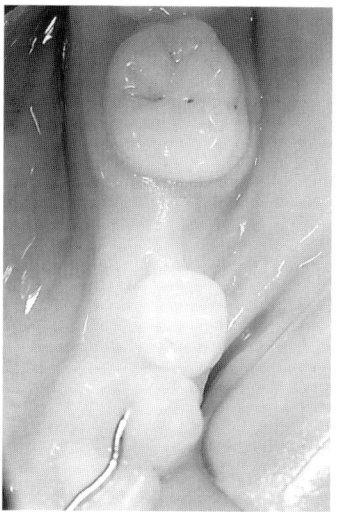

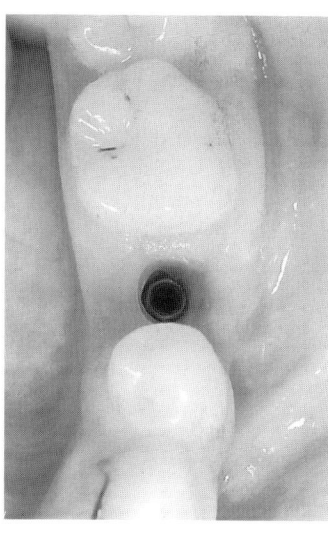

Fig. 7. The Final result. Occlusal view shows the advantage in terms of tooth preservation with this type of reconstruction.

Fig. 8. Male patient with congenitally missing 35. The buccal concavity in edentulous ridge is obvious.

Fig. 9. After implant placement and ridge augmentation.

ridge augmentation), surgery (e.g. axis of implant, papilla preservation) and abutment connection (e.g. combination with grafting procedures) and design of prosthetic superstructures, must be carefully planned and carried out.

In patients with high lip-lines, the aesthetic results with single tooth implants may be inferior to those obtained with FPDs.

Partially and completely edentulous patients

Few abutment teeth and unfavorable distribution within the jaw may be seen as indications for removable partial dentures (RPD).

The disadvantages of RPDs and full dentures are discussed below.

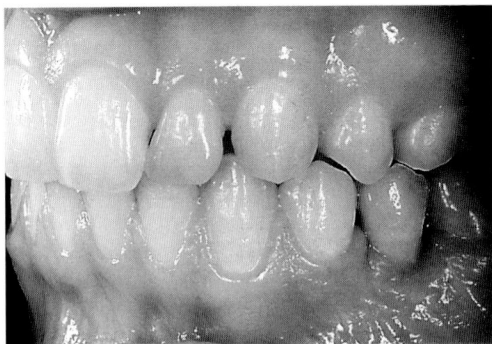

Fig. 10. Buccal view. Result of single tooth implant 35.

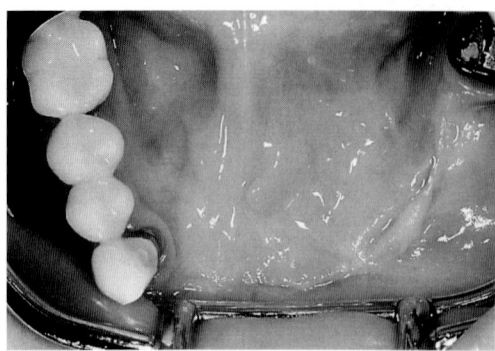

Fig. 11. Male patient (aged 32) with missing 42–36 as a result of a car accident. Rehabilitation with a conventional FPD is impossible.

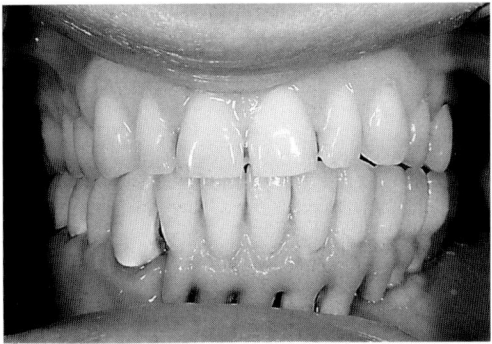

Fig. 12. Same patient after incorporation of seven implants and a porcelain–metal bridge. There are no visible metal parts.

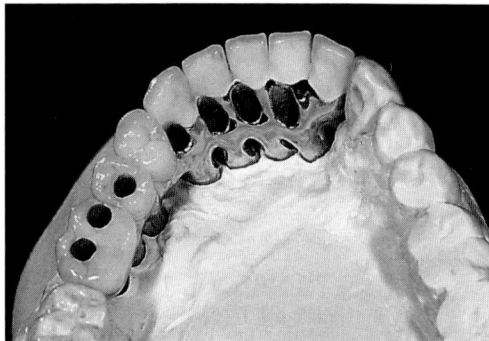

Fig. 13. Lingual view of the prosthesis. Screw access holes are in an optimal position, because implant directions were planned prior to surgery.

Comfort. It is often necessary to cover the palate with a palatal strap in order to enhance base extension and to give greater rigidity. Tongue space may be narrowed by a lingual bar, and a full denture covers even more oral tissue.

Psychology. At each removal, an RPD will always remind the wearer of his/her disturbed physical integrity, and this may result in psychological problems. Today, in patients with severe or complete tooth loss, which previously could only be restored with RPDs or full dentures, implants are the only solution for a fixed restoration.

Maintenance. Plaque accumulation is increased in the presence of RPDs. This disadvantage can only be minimized by strict oral and denture hygiene. The smooth titanium or glazed porcelain surface of an implant-supported prosthesis seems to accumulate less plaque. This may be of particular importance in elderly patients, where plaque control can be very difficult.

Costs. An RPD or a full denture may be the most economical alternative.

Surgery

The basic criteria for osseointegration are discussed below.

Diagnosis

Presurgical diagnosis is extremely important in order to evaluate bone quality and quantity, both of which have a great influence on the prognosis.

Injuries to vital structures such as the inferior alveolar nerve or the mental nerve can and must be avoided by means of radiographs (e.g. panoramic films, CT-scans). The prosthetic goals must be known to the surgeon, since integrated but improperly placed implants may produce an unacceptable final result.

Infection control

Surgery must be performed under strictly sterile conditions. Osseointegration will not take place in infected implant sites.

Surgical technique

Implant bed preparation must be carried out as gently as possible, because trauma to bone tissue will lead to the development of poorly differentiated scar tissue (*Eriksson* 1984)[21]. Initial stability also appears to be vital for osseointegration.

Soft tissue management

Gentle treatment of the soft tissues (e.g. papilla preservation) will prevent aesthetic failures.

Unfavourable implant sites

Difficult implant placement sites are also very frequent, especially in the case of missing posterior teeth. In the upper jaw, implant placement may interfere with a low sinus, in the lower jaw with the inferior alveolar nerve. Site development procedures in such situations are discussed below.

Sinus elevation. A surgical procedure may be carried out to elevate the membranous floor of the sinus cavity by separating it from its inferior and lateral connections. The space is then filled with bone or biomaterials, usually with the simultaneous insertion of implants, in order to gain vertical bone height.

Bone grafting. Iliac bone grafting procedures have also been used to achieve greater vertical height[24].

Nerve repositioning

Inferior alveolar nerve repositioning procedures which allow use of the full thickness of the mandible have also been proposed. However, although these techniques show promising early results, long-term results are not yet available.

The surgical procedures described above are not without risk, so the development of implant designs, which can be used even in resorbed jaws remains a challenge for the future.

Aesthetics. Gingiva around titanium abutments often looks dark, like gingiva around non-vital discolored roots. From a biological point of view, titanium may be the most suitable material subgingivally, but for aesthetic reasons tooth-coloured abutments

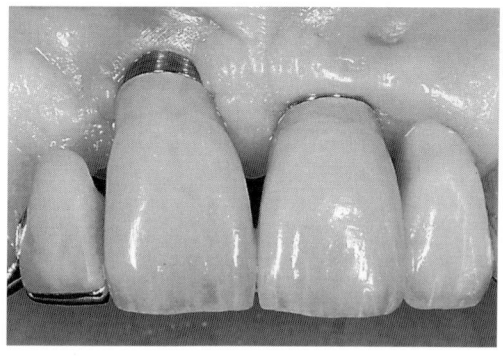

Fig. 14. Soft tissue recession around an implant at 11. The implant is osseointegrated, but from an aesthetic point of view it must be called as failure.

with similar light transmission properties to those of vital roots might be more desirable.

Outlook for the future

Long-term studies

Most manufacturers and users of implant systems have yet to present adequate follow-up studies and long-term results. Statistics concerning actual survival rates must cover extended periods, in order to be clinically significant. It is not only necessary to study the survival rates of implants and superstructures, but also the aesthetic long-term results (e.g. changes in soft tissue appearance).

Premarketing standards

It would be helpful to define and establish international premarketing standards for new implant systems or new designs, prior to their introduction onto the market.
These standards could be developed by universities, manufacturers and qualified dental practitioners.

Summary

With the constantly increasing demand for implant-supported restorations, the criteria for success for the three factors involved in implantology (dentist, implant system and patient) are evaluated. Treatment alternatives are presented, together with their advantages and disadvantages, and possible directions for future developments are discussed.

References

[1] Albrektsson, T., Brånemark, P.-I., Hansson, H. A. and Lindstrom, J. Osseointegrated titanium implants. Requirements for insuring a long-lasting direct bone-to-implant anchorage in man. Acta Orthop Scand 1981; 52: 155–170.

[2] Brånemark, P.-I. Osseointegration and its experimental background. J Prosthet Dent 1983; 50: 399–410.

[3] Carlsson, L., Rostlund, L., Albrektsson, B., Albrektsson, T., Brånemark, P.-I. Osseointegration of titanium implants. Acta Orthop Scand 1986; 57: 285–289.

[4] Blomberg, S., Lindquist, L. W. Psychological reactions to edentulousness and treatment with jawbone-anchored bridges. Acta Psychiatr Scand 1983; 68: 251–260.

[5] Greenfield, E. J. An artificial root. Dent Brief 1910; 15: 837–839.

[6] Brånemark, P.-I., Breine, U., Lundström, J., Adell, R., Hansson, B. O., Ohlsson, Å. Intra-osseous anchorage of dental prosthesis. 1. Experimental studies. Scand J Plast Reconstr Surg 1969; 3: 81–100.

[7] Brånemark, P.-I., Hansson, B. O., Adell, R. Osseo-integrated implants in the treatment of the edentulous jaw. Experience from a 10 year period. Scand J Plast Reconstr Surg 1977; 16: 1–132.

[8] Albrektsson, T., Zarb, G., Worthington, D. P., Eriksson R.A. The long-term efficacy of currently used dental implants: A review and proposed criteria of success. Int J Oral Maxillofac Implants 1986; 1: 11–25.

[9] Albrektsson, T., Sennerby, L. Direkte Knochenveran-kerung von oralen Implantaten: Klinische und experimentelle Betrachtungen des Konzepts der Osseointegration. Parodontologie 1990; 4: 307–320.

[10] Obwegeser, H. Der atrophische Kiefer aus der Sicht des Kieferchirurgen. Schweiz Mschr Zahnheilk 1977; 87: 946.

[11] Albrektsson, T., Brånemark, P.-I., Hansson, H. A., Ivarsson, B., Jönsson. Ultrastructural analysis of the interface zone of titanium and gold implants. In: Clinical applications of biomaterials. Advances in Biomaterials (eds Lee, A. J. C., Albrektsson, T., Brånemark, P.-I.). John Wiley & Sons Ltd, pp. 167–177. Chichester, New York 1982.

[12] Albrektsson, T., Hansson, H. A., Ivarsson, B. Interface analysis of titanium and zirconium bone implants. Biomaterials 1985; 6: 97–101.

[13] Jarcho M. Biomaterial aspects of calcium phosphates. Properties and applications. Dent Clin North Am 1986; 30: 25–47.

[14] Thomas, K. A., Kay, J. F., Cook, S. D. Jarcho, M. The effect of surface macrotexture and hydroxylapatite coating on the mechanical strengths and histologic profiles of titanium implant materials. J Biomed Mater Res 1987; 21: 1395–1414.

[15] Maniatopopulos, C., Pilliar, R. M., Smith, D. C. Threaded versus porous surfaced designs for implant stabilization in bone endodontic implant model. J Biomed Mater Res 1986; 20: 1309–1333.

[16] Skalak, R. Biomechanical considerations in osseointegrated prosthesis. J Prosthet Dent 1983; 49: 843–848.

[17] Buser, D., Schenk, R. K., Steinemann, S., Fiorellini, J. P., Fox, C. H., Stich, H. Influence of surface characteristics on bone integration of titanium implants. A histomorphometric study in miniature pigs. J Biomed Mater Res 1991; 25: 889–902.

[18] Brånemark, P.-I. Introduction to osseointegration. In: Tissue integrated prostheses. Osseointegration in clinical dentistry (eds Brånemark, P.-I., Zarb, G., Albrektsson, T.), pp. 1–76. Berlin: Quintessence, 1985.

[19] Schroeder, A., Sutter, F., and Krekeler, G. Orale Implantologie. Allgemeine Grundlagen und ITI Hohlzylindersystem. Stuttgart, Georg Thieme, 1988.

[20] Carlsson, L., Rostlund, T., Albrektsson, B., et al. Implant fixation improved by close fit. Acta Orthop Scand 1988; 59: 272–275.

[21] Eriksson, R. A. Heat induced bone tissue injury. An in vivo investigation of heat tolerance of bone tissue and temperature rise in the drilling of cortical bone (Thesis). Göteborg, Sweden: University of Gothenburg, 1984.

[22] Kasemo, B., Lausmaa, J. Surface science aspects of inorganic biomaterials. CRC Crit Rev Clin Neurobiol 1986; 2: 335–380.

[23] Albrektsson, T., Zarb, G., Worthington, P., Eriksson, A. R. The long-term efficacy of currently used dental implants: A review and proposed criteria of success. Int J Oral Maxillofac Implants 1986; 1: 11–25.

[24] Keller, E. E., Van Roekel, N. B., Desjardins, R. P., et al. Prosthetic-surgical reconstruction of the severely resorbed maxilla with illiac bone grafting and tissue-integrated prosthesis. Int J Oral Maxillofac Implants 1987; 2: 155–165.

Chapter 2

Treatment modalities for prosthetic rehabilitation in patients with full and partial edentulism

P. Battistuzzi

Partial edentulism may occur in many forms. The simple mutilation arises when a few teeth, or parts of a tooth, are missing; more complicated situations involve the loss of more teeth and also alveolar bone. In the past many attempts have been made to classify partial edentulism according to certain criteria. A useful classification is that proposed by Eichner[1] (Fig. 1). This is based on the presence of a number of supporting areas. The supporting areas in the dentition are important for oral function. This means that in therapeutic selection, the condition of the supporting areas and the functioning of the masticatory system must be taken into account. In addition to the functional criteria, the quality of the remaining dentition plays a role. There is a distinction between simple dental mutilations and complex dental mutilations. In the first instance, the defect is the only anomaly, while in the second case, in addition to the defect, other problems, complicating factors, are present. These may be:

(1) Inadequate motivation, neglect;
(2) Caries;
(3) Periodontal breakdown;
(4) Migrations;
(5) Orthodontic abnormalities;
(6) Craniomandibular dysfunction.

These complicating factors are sometimes the cause of the mutilation (for example through caries) or the result (for example through migration). It is also possible that there is no cause-and-effect relationship as in orthodontic disorders (for example Angle Class 2, II), where restorative treatment could be hampered.

During treatment planning, we try to eliminate the complicating factors and to control them. This takes place during the preliminary phase of the treatment.

In the case of lost teeth, the force distribution in the masticatory apparatus is disturbed. The consequences depend upon the influence of several general and local factors, including:

(1) Age of the patient
(2) Number of lost teeth
(3) Periodontal condition
(4) Interdigitation/position of the tongue, position of cheeks and lips
(5) Adaptability/neuromuscular tolerance.

The influence of these factors may be positive as well as negative (Fig. 2). The morphological and functional changes may be regarded as either adaptations to the changed circumstances, or else as pathological changes. It may be stated that the

A1
A2
A3
B1
B2
B3
C1
C2
C2
C3

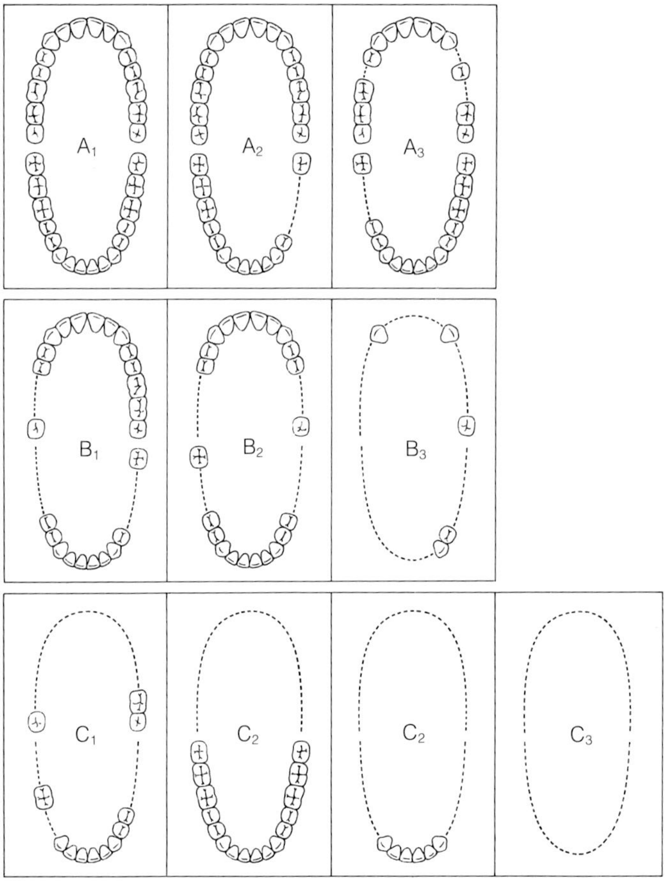

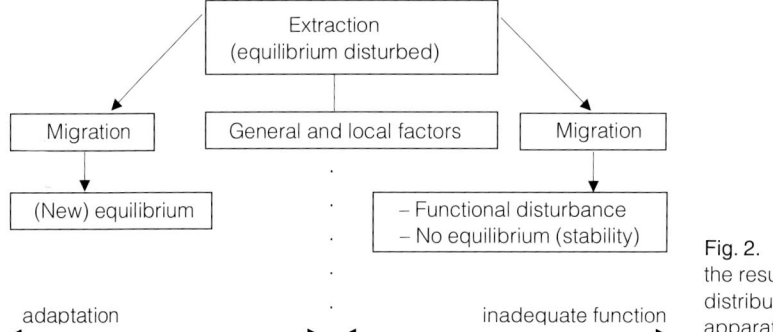

Add. A_{1-2-3}

Add. B_{1-2-3}

Add. C_{1-2-3}

Fig. 1. Classification according to *Eichner*[1].
A = antagonistic contact in all four supporting areas;
B = antagonistic contact in less than four contact areas;
C = antagonistic contact absent.

Extraction
(equilibrium disturbed)
Migration
General and local factors
Migration
(New) equilibrium
– Functional disturbance
– No equilibrium (stability)
adaptation
inadequate function

Fig. 2. Schematic representation of the results of extractions upon force distribution in the masticatory apparatus.

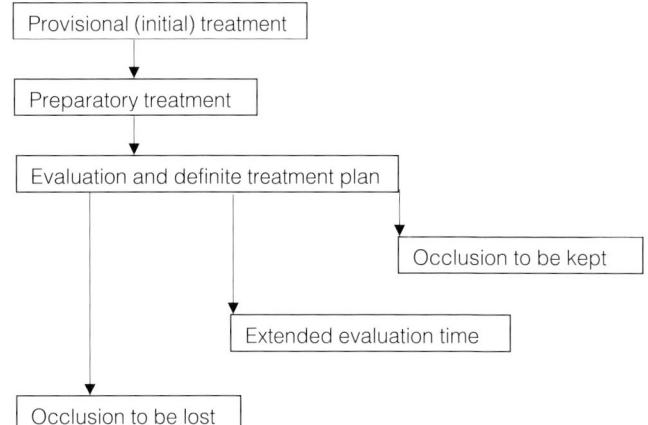

Fig. 3. Scheme to be applied in occlusal therapy

consequences of missing teeth may vary from individual to individual, and are difficult to predict.

For the patient, aesthetics are often the most important consideration and motivates him/her to seek dental help. If adaptation leads to an acceptable situation, there should be a reluctance of the practitioner to seek prosthetic treatment.

General treatment philosophy

The primary goal of clinical dentistry is to maintain the functional dentition for life. In this respect, there are still insufficient data to indicate how this objective may be achieved. On the contrary, there are a number of frequently contradictory therapeutic solutions. *Pilot*[2] formulated two partly connected reasons to justify certain types of treatment:

(1) The dental practitioner has scientific evidence that treatment is necessary in order to restore essential function and prevent predictable damage.

(2) The patient wishes to undergo the treatment. If scientific evidence is available, treatment should be based on this.

In many situations, objective guidelines are not available. It is therefore advisable only to carry out treatment or to use prosthetic appliances with obvious advantages. This should be balanced by avoiding therapies which involve certain risks. The following points should be taken into account:

(1) Missing teeth do not always need to be replaced;

(2) Perform only the treatment necessary to solve the relevant problems (problem-oriented diagnosis and treatment planning);

(3) If teeth are to be restored or replaced, first eliminate the complicating factors. This means that the treatment is carried out in stages, and the preliminary treatment evaluated on completion;

(4) In order to reduce the damage due to restorative procedures and to increase the predictability of the outcome, treatment should be of high level and as atraumatic as possible;

(5) After completion of the treatment, the

patient is placed on a recall and maintenance system, with frequency dependent on the individual needs of the patient.

In order to set up a well-founded treatment plan, a long period of observation of the patient is needed. The treatment should start with a provisional plan, which is tested and modified during the initial phase (Fig. 3). Only after evaluation of the initial treatment, should one proceed to the definitive treatment.

An important factor is the prognosis for the remaining dentition. If this is good, then one can aim for permanent maintenance and rehabilitation of the occlusion. If it is possible, crown and bridgework is preferable. If the prognosis is poor, then the remaining occlusion will be lost. The gradual disintegration may be delayed through a series of measures, the object of which is to preserve the alveolar process.

If the prognosis is uncertain, then the preparatory (initial) treatment phase should be extended and evaluation postponed to a later stage.

Standard solutions

General remarks

The so-called standard solutions include all the standard treatments in cases of mutilations and functional problems. From the range of possible solutions, the best possibility is chosen, based on the specific situation and the wishes of the patient. The standard solutions should be formulated according to the starting points as set out below.

The beneficial aspects of prosthetic care play an important role in this respect. *Fröhlich* and *Körber*[3] studied the benefits of different prosthetic treatment modalities in a number of cases of partial edentulism. The following criteria were taken into account: the number of years the patient had functioned satisfactorily with the prosthetic appliance, the presence of occlusal disturbances, and the mobility of the abutment teeth. The authors came to the following conclusions:

(1) The benefits of the treatment are greatly influenced by the number of abutment teeth and their position in the dental arch;

(2) The benefits are greatest in cases where the prosthesis is fully supported by the teeth;

(3) If the number of abutment teeth is sufficient and they are favourably situated, the benefit in the case of a tooth- and mucosa-supported prosthesis is relatively high;

(4) In cases of extensive dental mutilation, where the abutment teeth are unfavourably positioned in the dental arch, the mucosa-supported prosthesis seems to provide a greater benefit than a tooth- and mucosa-supported prosthesis;

(5) In cases where there are only a few remaining teeth, overdentures are relatively successful.

The survival rate of metal cast, removable partial dentures is 75% after 5 years and 50% after 10 years[4] (See chapter 3).

Hedegård[5] considered variable alveolar bone height and plaque levels to be of great importance in the choice between removable partial dentures (RPD) and fixed partial dentures (FPD). On the basis of clinical research he concluded that:

(1) When sufficient alveolar bone height and optimal oral hygiene are present, there is a wide choice of treatment possibilities;

(2) Should oral hygiene not be adequate, FPD seems to cause less iatrogenic damage than RPD;

(3) If alveolar bone height is reduced, but there is good oral hygiene, an FPD is preferable;

(4) If oral hygiene is inadequate, the prosthetic treatment should be regarded as an intermediate stage, leading to an overdenture or a complete denture.

The results obtained with recent prosthetic developments such as adhesive bridgework and the attachment of prosthetic appliances to implants are noteworthy. The survival rate of adhesive bridges in the anterior region over 10 years is 50%, but it is expected that the failure rate will decrease with technical improvements.

The low failure rates of FPD supported by osseointegrated implants in edentulous patients are well known[6]. In partially edentulous patients the results in the short term are comparable with those in fully edentulous patients. The failure rates related to the maxilla and mandible are; respectively; 5.7% and 6.5%[7]. The results with overdentures on implants are also very promising, although the failure rate is related to the type of implant and the condition of the jaw.

Presenting problems

In choosing standard solutions the following distinctions regarding the mutilation in the dentition are useful:

(1) Interrupted dental arch;
(2) Shortened dental arch;
(3) Edentulous jaw against partially dentate jaw;
(4) Edentulous upper and lower jaw.

Interrupted dental arch

Interrupted dental arches occur in many forms. From epidemiological studies it is to be expected that interruptions occur frequently in the molar and premolar area, particularly in the lower jaw. The need for treatment in such cases depends upon the degree of aesthetic disturbance, discomfort during chewing and the level of mandibular stability. When no occlusal disturbances occur after prolonged observation, replacement can be omitted.

The following possibilities may be considered:

(1) No treatment (Fig. 4);
(2) Orthodontic closure of the space;
(3) Autotransplantation;
(4) Tooth-supported appliance.

   (i) Fixed
     (a) FPD
     (b) adhesive bridgework

   (ii) Removable
     (a) RPD
     (b) RPD with (semi) precision attachment
     (c) RPD with adhesive attachment

(5) Implant-supported appliance

   (i) Supported on implants
     (a) crown
     (b) FPD

   (ii) Supported on implants and natural teeth
     (a) crown
     (b) FPD
     (c) RPD

(6) Mucosa-supported appliance
     (a) acrylic resin (interim) RPD.

Interrrupted dental arch

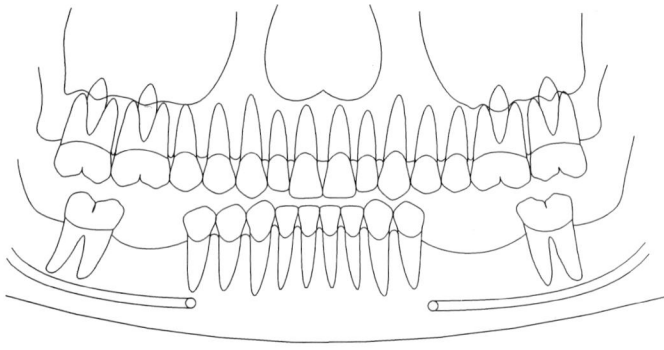

Fig. 4. No treatment needed because no harmful changes occurred and adaptation has led to an acceptable situation for the patient.

Shortened dental arch

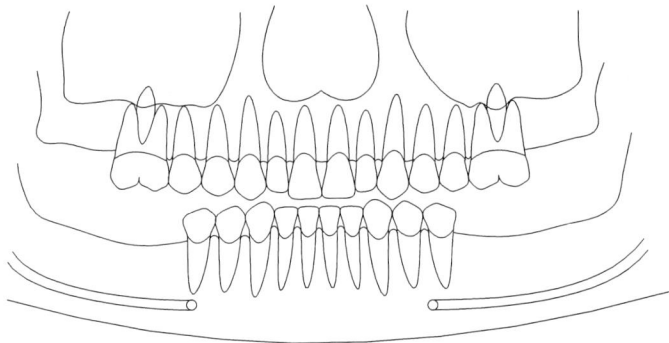

Fig. 5. No treatment needed because no harmful changes occurred and adaptation has led to an acceptable situation for the patient.

Shortened dental arch

Owing to the absence of posterior teeth, vertical dimension can decrease and there may be increased occlusal load in the anterior region.

Owing to loss of occlusal support, changes in the position of the condyle in the temporomandibular joint may take place. The masticatory efficiency is decreased, but in cases of symmetrical shortening up to the second premolar, masticatory function remains adequate. Adaptation to the changed circumstance occurs and gives rise to a new stable situation. The need for treatment of the shortened dental arch depends primarily on aesthetic appearance, chewing comfort and mandibular stability. Extension of a shortened dental arch is only useful in cases where relevant problems can be solved.

Several possibilities may be considered for a shortened dental arch:

(1) No treatment (Fig. 5);
(2) Tooth-supported appliance
   (i) adhesive bridgework
   (ii) FPD (Fig. 6);
(3) Tooth- or mucosa-supported appliances
   (i) RPD (Fig. 7)
   (ii) RPD (semi) precision attachment
   (iii) RPD with adhesive attachment

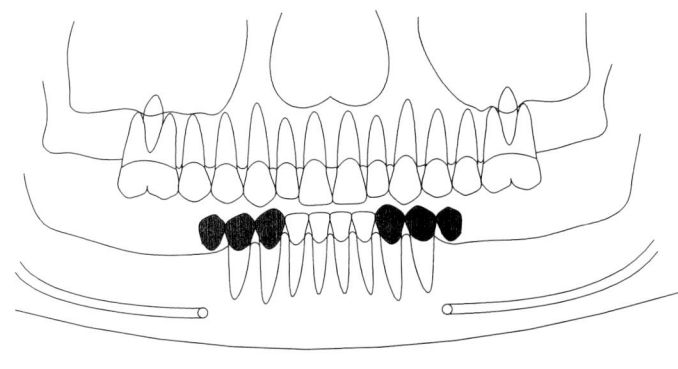

Fig. 6. Tooth-supported appliance (FPD).

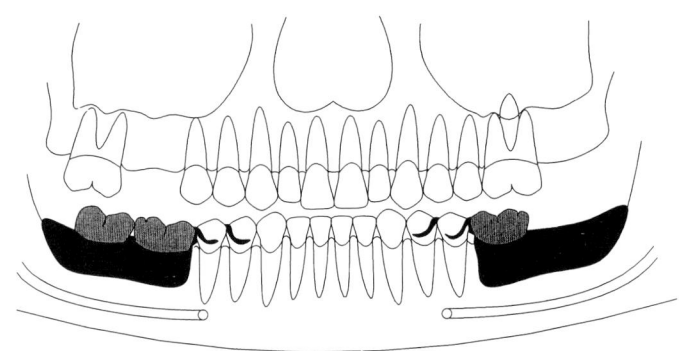

Fig. 7. Distal free-end removable partial denture (RPD). There is a high risk of bone resorption under the saddles since the latter are not distally tooth-supported. The abutment teeth are more prone to caries and periodontal problems if optimal plaque control is not maintained .

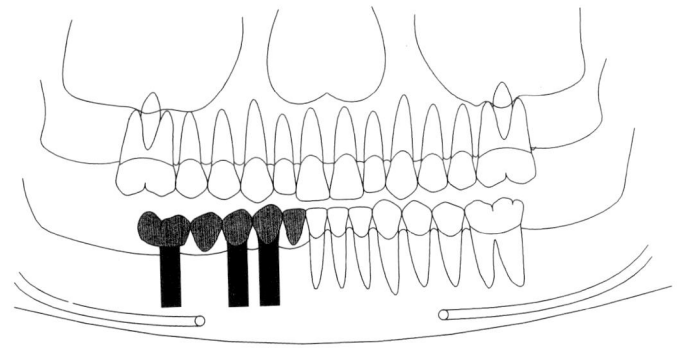

Fig. 8. Implant-supported fixed prosthesis.

(4) Implant-supported appliance
    (i) Supported on implants
        (a) crown
        (b) FPD (Fig. 8)
    (ii) Supported on implants and natural
         teeth

        (a) crown
        (b) FPD
        (c) RPD
(5) Mucosa-supported appliance
    (i)   acrylic resin (interim) RPD.

Edentulous jaw opposing partially dentate jaw

The mutilation pattern usually consists of an edentulous upper jaw opposing a (partially) dentate lower jaw. In addition to the replacement of the upper dentition, the occlusion must be restored and maintained in bilateral balance. Loading in the upper anterior region must be avoided. Solutions to the partially edentulous jaw were discussed earlier. If, in spite of taking all the necessary precautions to achieve a bilaterally balanced occlusion, good function is not achieved, the placement of implants in the edentulous jaw should be considered. The prosthetic reconstruction may involve either an FPD or an overdenture with a (semi) precision attachment.

Edentulous upper and lower jaw

Patients who have problems with complete dentures are roughly divided into two groups. The first group consists of patients with extensive problems of acceptance of the edentulous state. This group may benefit from the provision of implants supporting an FPD in the upper and lower jaws. The second group consists of patients with retention problems. This occurs particularly with lower dentures. In contrast to the patients in the first group, this group will accept a removable appliance. In such cases; the same solutions apply as discussed in the previous section. If only one jaw is provided with implants, there is a danger that the retention problem may be transferred to the opposing edentulous jaw.

Conclusions

In this chapter the importance of treatment planning and of distinguishing between simple and complex dental mutilations are discussed. Neglect of the dentition results in caries and periodontitis, which are the primary causes of the natural breakdown of the dentition. The life-span of the more commonly used prosthetic appliances is considered. Finally, the mutilation patterns of an interrupted dental arch, a shortened dental arch, an edentulous jaw against a dentate jaw and edentulous upper and lower jaws are discussed.

References

[1] Eichner, K. Gruppeneinteilung des Lückengebisses. Dtsch Zahnärztl Z 1955; 10: 1831–1834.

[2] Pilot, T. Pleidooi tegen het verlengen van de verkorte tandboog. Ned Tijdschr Tandheelkd 1978; 85: 477–480.

[3] Fröhlich, E., Körber, E. Die prothetische Versorgung des Lückengebisses. Befunderhebung und Planung. 2. Auflage. München: Carl Hansen Verlag, 1977.

[4] Vermeulen, A. H. B. M. De partiële prothese. Een decennium klinische evaluatie. Proefschrift: Nijmegen, 1984.

[5] Hedegård, B. Reduziert festsitzender oder herausnehmbarer Zahnersatz in parodontal behandelten Gebisstendenzen. ZWR 1979; 88: 772–775.

[6] Adell, R., Lekholm, U., Rockler, B., Brånemark, P.-I. A 15-year study of osseointegrated implants in the treatment of the edentulous jaw. Int J Oral Surg 1981; 10: 387–416.

[7] Naert, I. The influence of prosthetic design and implant type on tissue reactions around oral implants (Thesis). Acta Biomedica Lovaniensia, 40. 1991.

Chapter 3

Longterm prognosis of conventional prosthodontic restorations

Th. Kerschbaum

Significance of treatment evaluation

A fixed or removable prosthodontic restoration should function well over a long period of time. On the one hand this shows the longevity of prosthodontic restorations; on the other hand many problems arise through evaluating treatment over such a long time span. Therefore, systematic follow-up studies and patient recalls are important means of assessment. No clinician should rely on "clinical impressions" a decade or more after the initial treatment. However, tracing patients after such a long time is also often a difficult logistic problem, which may lead to non-representative samples yielding false statistical results. Their general applicability may therefore be in doubt.

The reasons for analysing the therapeutic success of prosthodontic treatments are best summarized under two fundamental concepts:

(1) Unsuccessful prosthodontic restorations may have important medical, dental, social, psychological, economic, or forensic consequences. For patients, failure means complaints, pain, and waste of both time and money. They may lose confidence in dental therapy. The clinician may lose job satisfaction and be disappointed in the work. In addition, short survival times of dental restorations have very important consequences with regard to health insurance systems. Economy in health care becomes especially relevant, when, in certain situations functionally equivalent treatments differ considerably in terms of expense.

Scientific clinical research is the only acceptable basis for assessing prosthodontic therapy. The importance of quality assurance is increasingly being discussed. Nowadays, inadequate dental treatments are successfully prosecuted in court.

(2) Analysing success and failure in prosthodontics helps to define indications, modify the therapeutic approach and improve the quality of dental materials. Medical and dental treatment is based on experience. Progress in these sciences is often the result of trial and error. Only through the critical evaluation of therapeutic results (Fig. 1) can this process continue.

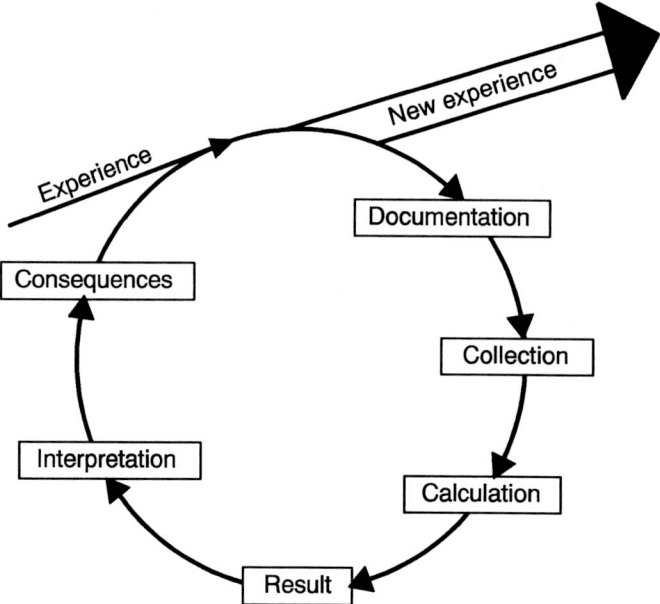

Fig. 1. Monitoring process of dental restorations (modified from *Scheibe* (1975).

Importance and meaning of study design

In general, the value of follow-up studies in prosthodontics is overestimated because many clinicians derive their therapeutic concepts mainly from retrospective (case control) trials. Follow-up studies are very useful in describing the adverse effects of therapeutic measures (monitoring, surveillance). They are far from ideal for comparing the results of different treatments, because they lack comparability, i.e. the structural, observational and representative conditions of the groups compared are not similar. Randomized (controlled) clinical trials are a standard method of evaluating treatment modalities. However, this type of study is not available in prosthodontics. Thus, case control studies remain our most important source of information on the long-term effects of fixed or removable pros-

theses. Nevertheless, one must be aware of the limitations.

Systematic recalls and follow-up studies in dentistry have a respectable tradition, especially in Europe. The Swiss prosthodontist *Dolder* stated 40 years ago that new prosthodontic treatments should be tried out on at least 50 patients and then observed for 3 to 5 years. Several dental material tests and technical experiments should also be carried out.

Determination of success and failure

Many authors have tried to answer the question "What is success or failure in prosthodontics?", without defining or creating standards of evaluation which are fully accepted by the profession. This problem will remain unsolved because of the many

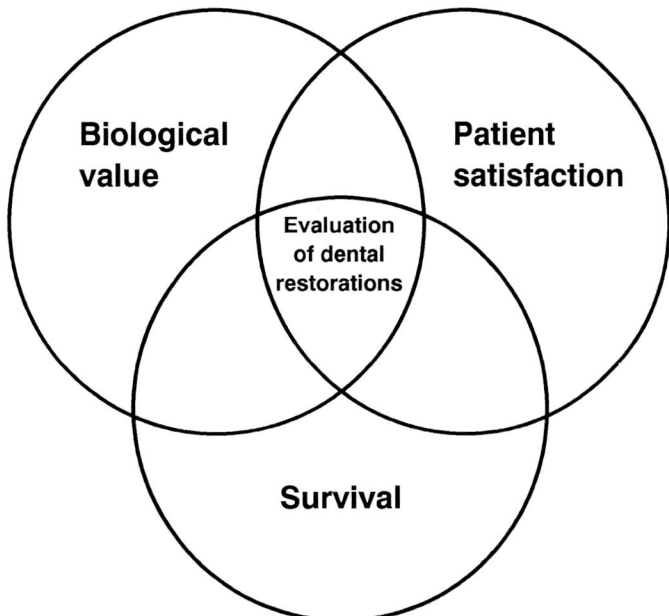

Fig. 2. The combination of three factors contributing to clinical evaluation of prosthodontic restorations.

biological, psychosocial, functional, technical, and construction factors which influence the "success" of crown and bridgework or a partial/complete denture. The phrase "a prosthesis functions well" ideally encompasses all these ideas, but has the same limitations as the term "success".

Consequently, very few studies use identical or even comparable criteria in their individual assessment. Owing to the lack of useful criteria, several parameters are recommended in this paper to describe success or failure in prosthodontics. Three main trends (Fig. 2) can be distinguished.

First, it is scientifically useful to analyse the occurrence or lack of unwanted side-effects caused by the treatment. Mainly, it is the **biological value** of the restoration, which is being estimated. The presence of periodontal or dysfunctional problems or secondary caries are used in longitudinal or cross-sectional studies. Follow-up treatment needs can be specified according to type involved and frequency of occurrence. In addition, technical failures (e.g. fractures, wear, corrosion, loss of aesthetics) may be observed, but many of these methods are not standardized, or only poorly so. It is frequently impossible to discriminate exactly between technical and biological failures, as can be demonstrated by the association between secondary caries and a crown's marginal gap. Thus, a clear cause-and-effect relationship cannot be verified. In many cases it is not known whether the observed secondary effects are due to the treatment or caused by the behaviour of the patient.

Secondly, with regard to cost factors, the period of function, or **survival-time**, of a restoration is critically important. Clinical experience shows that this period is the result of all the factors and injuries which influence functional survival time. The method underlines the significance of the time factor which is of the utmost importance in the dental profession. Dentists' perceptions of the longevity of dental restorations are influenced by beliefs about the effects of replacement and indications[1].

This type of information can be termed "hard" data because medical facts can be collected from patient records or registers (insurance companies, health services) where the data for each patient are collected over a long period. Unfortunately, it is a typical shortcoming of this method that the functional quality of the prosthesis and the reasons for failure cannot be evaluated. Finally, it is also useful to document the patient's degree of **acceptance and satisfaction. In general, more than 90% of patients are satisfied with their treatment. However, the fact that patients rarely have the opportunity to compare their treatment with the relevant alternatives should be taken into account.**

In summary, a combination of the three methods outlined above yields the most consistent assessment of a prosthodontic treatment, bearing in mind that comparisons with other treatments frequently lead to faulty results. Only longitudinal studies can give an exact insight into the longevity of restorations[2, 3]. Data should be collected for at least 5 years before a new prosthetic therapy can be recommended.

Results of long-term studies

Crowns and bridges

It has only recently been shown that the longevity and function of fixed dental restorations (crowns and bridgework) is much

greater than previously believed. The superior functional value of crowns and bridgework was known before, owing to:

(1) Excellent adaptation by patients, because they accept such restorations as their own teeth and not as "prostheses";
(2) Efficient chewing using periodontal support;
(3) Possibility of exact occlusal reconstruction;
(4) Limitation of possible adverse effects to the reconstructed area of the jaw (except occlusion);
(5) No compliance problems because patients cannot seat the restoration incorrectly.

The most important adverse effects can be listed as follows:

(1) Secondary caries at the margin of the crown preparation;
(2) Irreversible pulpal pathology owing to the preparation and subsequent procedures (liners, drying, cementation) leading to endodontic complications and periapical lesions;
(3) Periodontal complications owing to margin placement below the gingiva, poor reconstruction of interproximal contact areas, food impaction, overextended crown contours or inadequate pontic design;
(4) Poor aesthetics owing to discolored, worn or fractured crown veneering material;
(5) Occlusal interference;
(6) Danger of tooth or pontic fracture;
(7) Necessity of recementation and retreatment owing to poor retention;
(8) Other technical complications (fracture of soldered joints and materials).

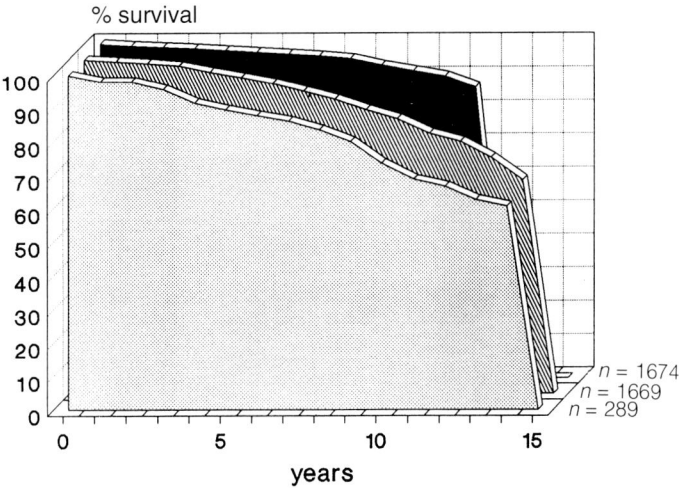

% survival

years

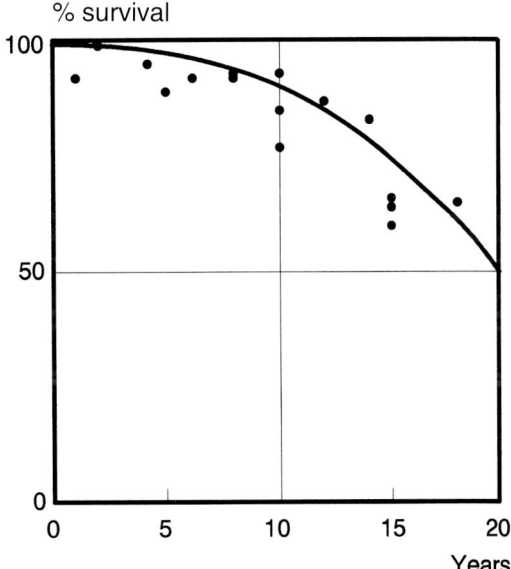

% survival

Years

Fig. 3. (a) Survival curves of bridges (*Leempoel*[5]. n = 1674, *Kerschbaum*[6]. n = 1669; *Erpenstein et al.*[7]. n = 298)
(b) Plotted data from Table I (except: *Roberts*, 1970).

Period of service

Systematic studies on the survival times of single crowns and bridges in large populations[4-7] show that satisfactory results were reported (Figs 3a, b and 4). Generally, failures of 5%, 10% and 40% after 5, 10 and 15 years, respectively, were reported. The median survival time of fixed cast metal and porcelain fused to metal (PFM) restorations

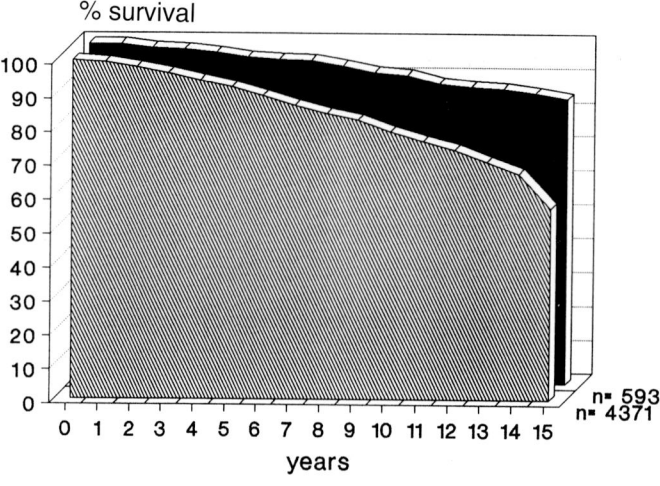

Fig. 4. Survival curves of single crowns (*Kerschbaum*[6]. n = 4371; *Erpenstein*[7]. n = 593).

Table I.   Results of longitudinal studies on survival of bridges; *n* = number of studied bridges/units/abutments

Year	Authors	*n*	Results of the study
1956	Morrant	122	after 1 year; 8% failure
1968	Kantorowicz	149	after 1–10 years; 15% failure
1970	Roberts (a)	1046	full crowns: 0.5% failure/year
			partial crowns: 1.7% failure/year
			post crowns: 4.4% failure/year
1970	Roberts (b)	1045	patients aged 16–20: 6.4% failure/year
			patients aged 21–35: 4.8% failure/year
			patients older than 35: 2.6% failure/year
1979	Nyman & Lindhe	332	after 6.2 years; 8% failure
1979	Rüeger	353	after 18 years; 35% lost (c&b)
1984	Reuter & Brose	121	failures from 1.5% to 2.9%/year
1986	Karlsson	1606	after 10 years; 93.3% in function
1987	Kerschbaum & Gaa	1666	after 8 years; 92.6% survival
1987	Leempoel	1674	after 12 years; 87% survival
1988	Georg et al.	504	after 2 years; 2.7% remade
1988	Pape	385	after 50 months; 95% survival
1988	Ödmann & Karlsson	100	after 8 years; 7% removed
1989	Karlsson	140	after 14 years; 17% lost
1991	Kerschbaum et al.	1073	after 15 years; 64% (±3%) survival
1992	Erpenstein et al.	298	after 15 years; 60% (±9%) survival

From *Kerschbaum* and *Leempoel*, 1989, updated).

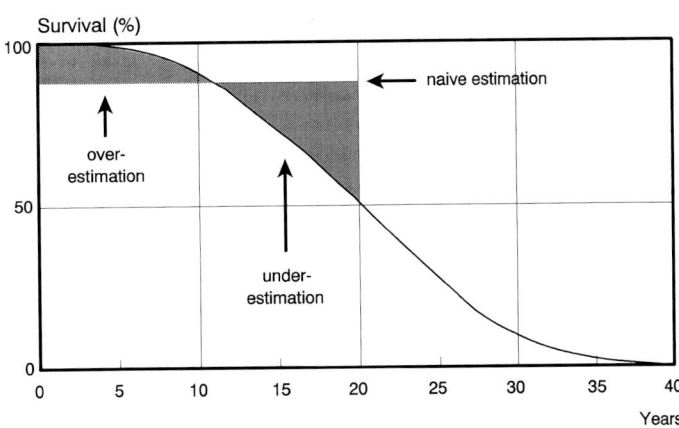

Fig. 5. Hypothetical survival curve for dental restorations: The Kaplan-Meier curve is an estimation of survival. For each year on the x-axis there is a probability on the y-axis that the restoration will remain in function at least *n* years. A short time after insertion (point zero) the loss of restorations is low; survival rates change with time and cannot be estimated as constant rates. This method of "naive estimation" overestimates early failures and underestimates late losses.

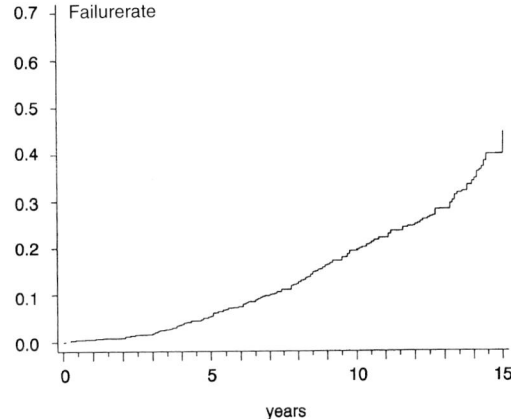

Fig. 6. Empirical cumulative hazard curve (example from *Kerschbaum*[6]) for bridges. In the first years after placement there is a very low risk of losing the bridge (0.8%/year). This increases to 2.7% per year 10 years after insertion (values calculated from the data). Data were available up to 15 years.

A plot of the empirical cumulative hazard curve visualizes time-dependent changes in the level of risk more precisely than the Kaplan-Meier survival curve, e.g. assuming a constant failure risk; in time the hazard curve will be approx. linear, whereas the Kaplan-Meier curve appears as a negative exponential. In practice, the first parts of both curves often seem to be reflections of each other, but differences increase over time.

is estimated at 20 years, based on follow-up studies of patients over 15 years. These results would therefore appear to be highly reliable.

Reasons for failures

Initial failures with crown and bridgework are very rare (about 1% per year) with an **increasing risk** as time progresses. Adequate statistical procedures, the Kaplan-Meier survival curves (Fig. 5) and the description of risk (hazard curve; Fig. 6), prove that there is no linear relationship between time and failure. It is therefore incorrect to describe failures in terms of constant rates per year (compare previous studies in Table I). It is possible that continuously acting, harmful influences are responsible for this development, whilst a high initial failure rate is due to inadequate case selection and poor treatment. Figure 7 shows the typical causes of failure of a restoration at different time intervals. The reasons can be

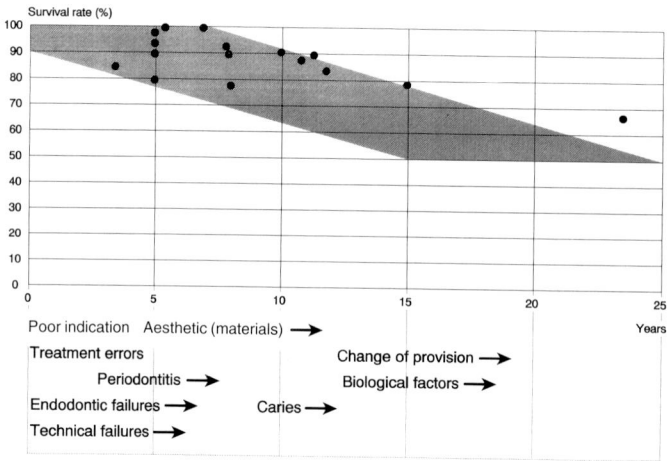

Fig. 7. Review of 16 studies and main reasons for loss of function related to the time intervals after insertion.

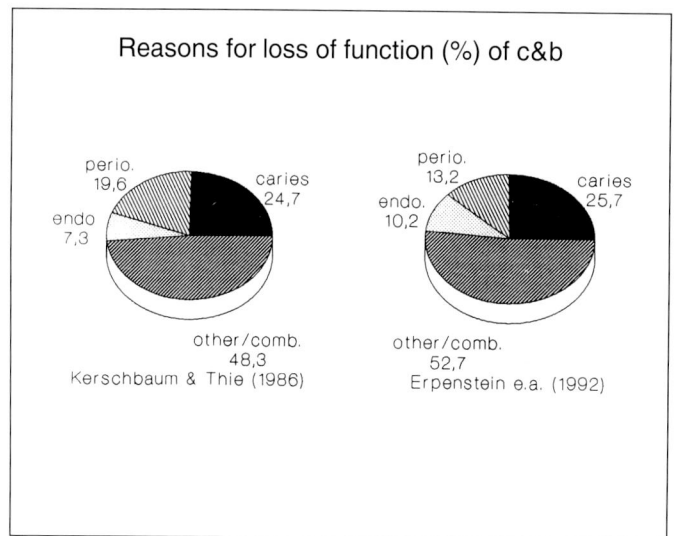

Fig. 8. Frequency distribution of reasons for loss of function for dental restorations (from *Kerschbaum* and *Thie*[10] and *Erpenstein* et al, 1992).

divided into two groups of approximately equal size: diseases (caries, periodontal, endodontic and periapical problems) and technical problems, as shown 20 years ago[9] and confirmed years later[7, 10, 11] (Fig. 8). Table II summarizes the studies described by *Kerschbaum* and *Leempoel*[12]; listing important biological and technical complications in crown and bridge therapy 10 years after placement. There are significant differences between the various types of

crowns and abutments. The best survival times are found among the cast full metal- and porcelain fused to metal crowns. For partial crowns, life-span is reduced, especially if they are used as abutments. The shortest life-span is associated with all-ceramic crowns (jacket crowns). It is still uncertain whether single crowns or bridges have a better prognosis; because conflicting results have been reported.

The majority of studies describing the

Table II. Summary of important biological and technical complications in crown- and bridge-therapy, 10 years after placement

Complication	Frequency	
Biological complications		
extraction of tooth (abutment)	approx.	3 – 5%
apical periodontitis	approx.	5%
secondary caries (crown-margin)	approx.	10 – 20%
loss of vitality/sensitivity	approx.	10 – 15%
Technical complications		
fracture of pontic	approx.	1%
loss of retention (recementation)	approx.	5 – 10%
defects of PFM-crowns	approx.	5 – 8%
fractures of all-ceramic front-crown	approx.	10 – 15%

From *Kerschbaum* and *Leempoel*, 1989, updated).

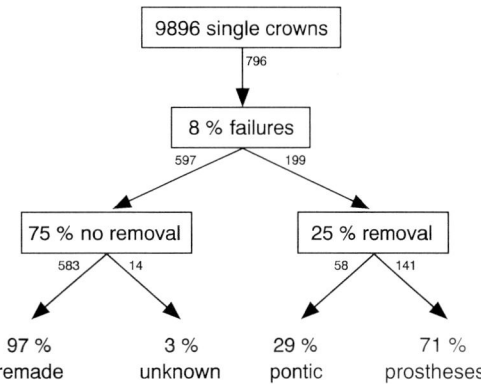

Fig. 9. Fate of 9896 single crowns related to type of retreatment (from *Kerschbaum* and *Leempoel*[12]). Removal = extractions of teeth; prosthesis = RPD or full denture.

Data from:
Leempoel (1988)

longevity of crown and bridgework clearly show that such restorations do survive for long periods. This fact has not yet been accepted worldwide. It is remarkable that even in failed cases, only a few patients are faced with abutment loss. Usually after failure, the restoration is renewed (Fig. 9). The belief that crown and bridgework contribute to the prolongation of the functional life of natural teeth is justified.

Removable partial dentures (RPD)

Period of service

The period of service of a cast metal frame prosthesis, today's treatment of choice in cases of extensive tooth loss, is significantly limited compared with fixed restorations. In

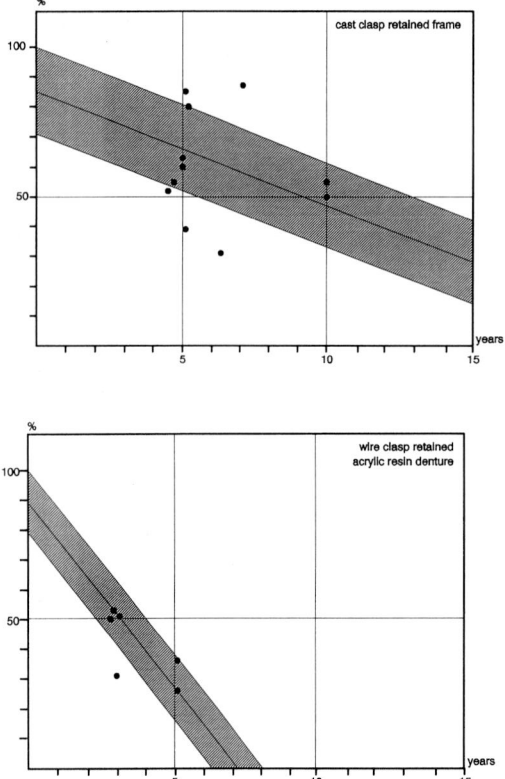

Fig. 10. Length of service of RPD-type (cast-clasp retained frame and wire-clasp retained acrylic resin denture base (from *Kerschbaum*[13]).

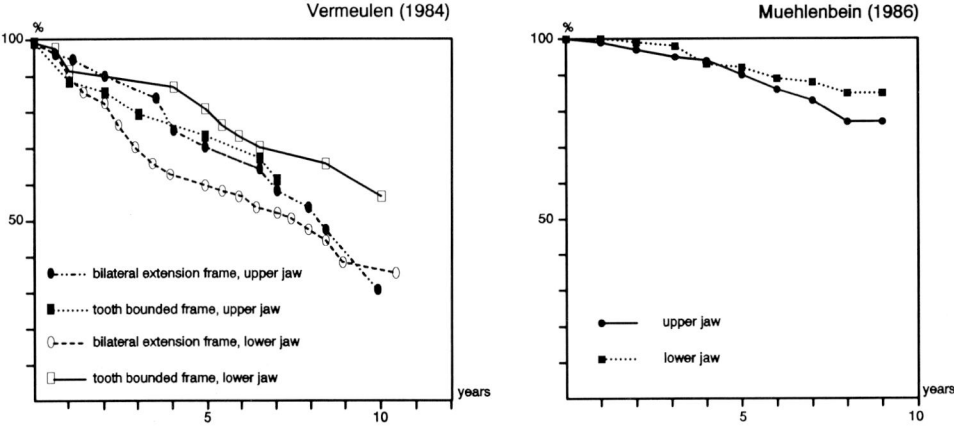

Fig. 11. Survival curves precision attachment retained RPDs (*Vermeulen*[14]; *Mühlenbein*[27]).

12 follow-up studies compiled by *Kerschbaum*[13] on cast-clasp-retained RPDs (Fig. 10) it was shown that the borderline of good clinical function was reached for 50% of the prostheses 6 to 10 years after insertion. A similar result was recorded for precision attachment-retained cast metal RPDs[14] (Fig. 11), while simple acrylic resin partial denture bases retained by wire clasps lasted about 3 years (Fig. 10). In addition to interim treatment, this last type of partial denture is not regarded as permanent prosthetic therapy. It is a fact that many RPDs are in situ for far too long (approx. 12 to 15 years) and frequently cause damage to the oral tissues.

About 85–90% of patients were satisfied with their RPDs. However, one should be aware of the fact that between 2 and 30% of Kennedy Class I RPDs were not worn. Among discontented patients, complaints about collection, retention or impaction of food, soreness and discomfort were most common.

Main reasons for loss of function

After insertion of the RPD, its interaction with oral hard and soft tissues is responsible for a number of important consequences. These can be divided into three groups; according to importance:

(1) Ecological changes in the oral cavity (plaque accumulation);
(2) Mechanical irritation and close contact of the RPD with the periodontium, oral mucosa and hard tissues;
(3) Non-physiological stress due to occlusal trauma and (horizontal) load.

Typical findings in clinical long-term studies of failed RPDs included caries, extractions, gingival recession, increased tooth mobility, changes in the oral mucosa, loss of alveolar bone; and functional disorders.

The most common results from studies with unsupervised usage of RPDs are discussed below (compiled from surveys by *Kerschbaum*[13].

Caries, extractions. Abutment teeth frequently developed caries and required extraction, especially if they were not crowned. Ten years post insertion, 5–13% of upper molars were removed for various reasons[14]. Approximately 50% of the abutment teeth; sound at the time of insertion, were filled, carious or removed 5 years after placement (patients who did not wear their RPD served as controls; the corresponding value was approximately 20%) (Fig. 12).

Caries on the surfaces of abutments was rarely observed to be in direct contact with clasps, but more frequently in the interproximal areas which contacted the denture saddle. Some lesions occurred in the cervical region between the clasp and the gingival margin. Extensive contact between parts of the RPD (lingual and upper plate design, continuous clasp) and hard tissues lead to decalcification or carious lesions. Prophylactic measures were tested in a small group and were effective[15–17], but patient compliance was poor.

Periodontitis. This was probably the most serious problem in RPD-wearers. The majority of follow-up studies indicated that inflammation, increased tooth mobility and a high number of periodontally involved teeth were registered. Only a few studies reported moderate or no pathological changes.

Lesions of the oral mucosa. Changes in the oral mucosa under saddles, major and minor connectors; were observed in one third of the cases within 5 years post

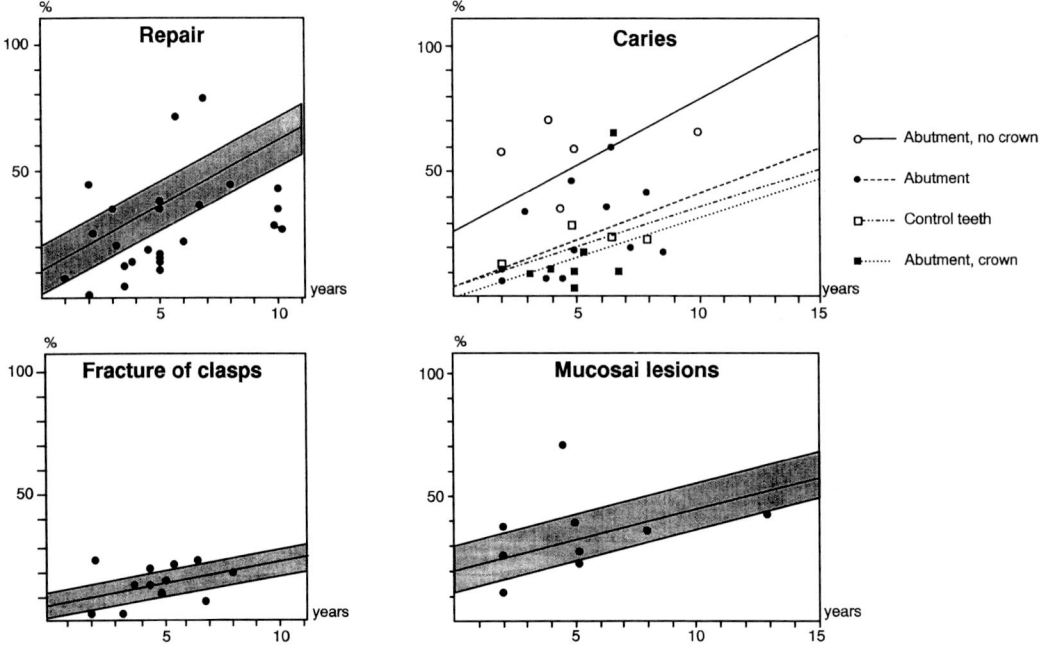

Fig. 12. Postinsertion treatment needs in RPDs (from *Kerschbaum*[13]). Need of repair, fractures of clasps, caries and secondary caries in abutments/non-abutments/control-teeth (RPD not worn) and mucosal lesions.

insertion (Fig. 12). These were due to impressions of connectors, traumatic injuries, uncontrolled sinking (in the case of free-end denture bases) and candidiasis resulting from poor oral hygiene.

Preservation of the alveolar ridge. One of the objectives in therapy with RPDs is the maintenance of alveolar bone in the edentulous areas. The two longitudinal studies by *Carlsson* et al.[18, 19] stated that free-end RPDs did not preserve alveolar bone. Clinical experience shows that bone loss is extensive if the RPD is not tooth-supported. Mucosa-born RPDs can cause extreme resorption.

Functional disorders. The reconstruction of an altered occlusion is a basic requirement of therapy with an RPD. After insertion of the RPD, muscle symptoms decreased, only to increase again to former levels after 6 months. Non-occlusion increased to 70% in double-extension RPDs after 2 years. In cases treated with telescopic attachments, occlusal stability was maintained longer than in cases treated with cast clasps[20, 21]. However, craniomandibular disorders in RPD-wearers were no more frequent than in other groups. About 90% of the patients with RPDs showed functional problems. There were no or only minor indications that the number of occlusal units was related to the frequency and severity of symptoms. Complete loss of occlusal units, even if limited to one quadrant, lead to functional limitations. An RPD should be the treatment of choice in cases of extremely shortened dental arches[22, 23].

Post insertion treatment needs. It is a common finding in longitudinal studies that cast metal frames are the type of prosthesis most likely to necessitate aftercare treatment (Fig. 12). Reports of fractures of clasps, connectors, and loss of retention of clasps are numerous. After 5 years, about 50% of the frame RPDs were relined, rebased or functionally re-established. Repair of the frame was necessary in more than one third of cases. Twenty per cent of the clasps or minor connectors were fractured, while 25% showed severe loss of retention.

Importance/validity of factors

The degree of tissue damage is influenced mainly by two factors: oral hygiene (professional recall, self-care) and denture design. The literature over the past 20 years shows that the prognosis for cases treated with a RPD depends more on the degree of plaque control and tissue tolerance than on construction of the prosthesis. It could be demonstrated in small groups of RPD-patients, that regular professional post-insertion care was effective if plaque control was good and the prosthesis was regularly checked[15, 24]. Thus, it can be concluded from the majority of the surveys, that "the wearing of an RPD per se does not cause dentogingival disease". However, the statement that "the risk of dentogingival disease appears higher in patients using a prosthesis than in patients who do not use one at all" is still valid[25]. This was reinforced by a comparative clinical trial of RPD versus fixed extension bridges[26]; which confirmed that treatment with distally extended cantilevered bridges was a more favourable alternative to treatment with RPDs in elderly patients.

Furthermore, the strict appliance of accepted design principles is necessary but not a guarantee of clinical success. Occlusal loading by tooth support (where loadable abutments are available) and periodontal relief of parts of the RPD seem to be essential criteria.

Full dentures and over-dentures

Period of service

Reliable data on the length of clinical service of full dentures and overdentures are scarce as compared to crown and bridge-work or RPDs. The reasons might be sought in the limited range of clinical concepts or methods, and the difficulty of evaluating the problems of complete denture wearers objectively. Important factors may also include the high mortality rate of the elderly and their poor attendance at recalls.

One survival study by *Mühlenbein*[27] followed up 509 upper and 205 lower full denture patients whose fees were paid by a private insurance company in Germany (Fig. 13). Five years after insertion, 81% (8 to 9 years: 67%) of the upper and 84% (8 to 9 years: 75%) of lower full dentures were still functioning. Retreatment needs were not significantly higher in mandibular dentures, although the difficulties relating to the anatomical situation and progressive resorption in the mandible are well known. A trend towards higher survival rates when comparing older (70 to 79 years) with younger patients was observed. This finding was interpreted as an adaption effect to the denture and was explained by the low level of consultation with the dentist. The period of

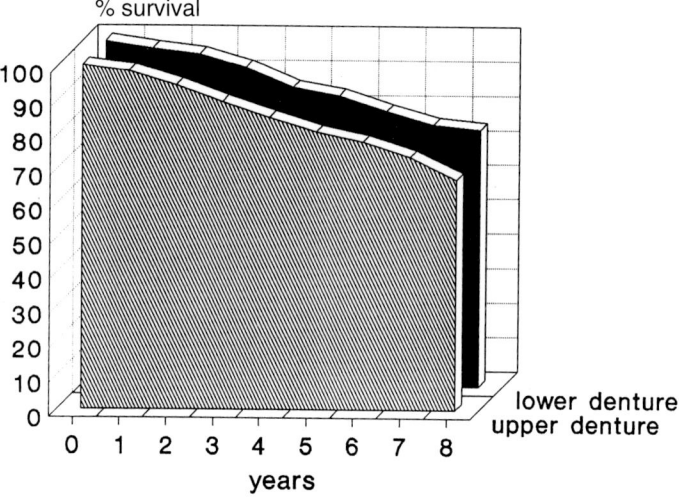

% survival

lower denture
upper denture

years

Fig. 13. Survival times for upper and lower full dentures, from *Mühlenbein*[27].

use of dentures was generally longer than either expected or desirable.

Evaluation of satisfaction and function

Subjective evaluations of fit, stability, retention, chewing ability and aesthetics of dentures are frequently used as important criteria in full denture patients. "Are you satisfied with your dentures?" is the most common question. The answers were reviewed by *Jonkman* and *Plooij*[28] (compiled from 47 studies). About 70% of patients answered "yes". Many dimensions of satisfaction (quality of the denture, condition of the oral structures, dentist–patient relationship, personality of the patient, influence of his/her socioeconomic level) were studied. *Carlsson's*[29] opinion was confirmed, that "no single factor appeared to determine the patients' satisfaction with his/her complete dentures".

As a rule there was little or no association between clinical success and satisfaction. In long-term studies, *Bergman* and *Carlsson*[30] found that more than half of the dentures needed renewal although the patients were satisfied. In 200 edentulous patients, *Dette* et al.[31, 32] confirmed that anatomical and physiological components were of minor importance in terms of satisfaction. Chewing ability, retention, stability of posterior teeth, relationship between the jaws and psychological variables were significant factors. The analysis of denture complaints confirmed that aesthetic problems dominated in the upper denture, whilst retention, stability and pain were the main problems of the lower denture[33].

Overdentures

Overdentures look similar to a full denture. The terms "cover-denture" and "hybrid prosthesis" are frequently used synonymously. In the simplest modification, retaining roots are covered with a prosthesis after restoring the root canal with amalgam. A

Table III. Overview of lost abutment teeth in six surveys of overdentures

Authors	A	B	C	D	E	F	G	H
No. of initial abutments:	59	23	52	233	14	54	70	679
Average years	13.5	2	5.5	5	2.5	5	6	9
No. of removed teeth	2	3	2	16	3	10	10	26
Percentage	3	13	4	7	21	19	14	4
Causes of removal:								
Periodontal	1	0	2	5	0	10	8	3
Caries	0	0	0	10	2	0	2	6
Endodontic	1	3	0	1	1	0	0	15
Fracture	0	0	0	0	0	0	0	2

A = *Fenton* and *Hahn*, 1978.   E = *Renner* et al., 1984.   From: *Jonkman* and *Plooij*, 1992.
B = *Davis* et al., 1981.   F = *Shaw*, 1984.
C = *Wabeke*, 1982.   G = *Lauciello* and *Ciancio*, 1985.
D = *Toolson* and *Smith*, 1983.   H = *Ettinger* and *Krell*, 1988.

more sophisticated method is to fix a hybrid prosthesis using cast-gold rootcaps with or without retention elements. A classical solution is the use of a Dolder-bar or a telescopic system as a retention device. The gold caps protect the teeth against caries for a long time[34].

Better denture retention and stability, improved chewing efficiency, reduced alveolar bone resorption and diminished mucosal load with overdentures lead to increased wearing comfort and better adaption. Disadvantages, especially for unprotected roots, were periodontal problems among abutments (plaque, bleeding, increased tooth mobility), endodontic failures, root caries (20–40% per year; see Table 3), extractions (4–21%), reduced aesthetics and a higher fracture risk to the base. Retreatment needs were estimated to be higher compared with full dentures.

Most of the clinical surveys concerning overdentures confirm the importance of ex-cellent oral and prosthesis hygiene. The patient is recommended to have regular inspections, but compliance with such a regimen is obviously poor.

Summary

The combination of the three methods of evaluation (biological effects, survival time, patient satisfaction) gives the most consistent view of the prognosis of a prosthodontic treatment.

The majority of the studies on the efficacy of crown and bridgework clearly show that this type of restoration should be characterized as a permanent or long-term restoration. The median lifetime is about 20 years. Compared with fixed restorations, the period of service of a cast metal frame prosthesis is shorter (about 10 years of service). The literature of the past 20 years shows that the prognosis for rehabilitation with an RPD depends more on the degree of plaque control than on design factors of the RPD. Patient satisfaction is reduced to 85–90%.

Reliable data on the length of clinical service of full dentures and overdentures are scarce. It is estimated to be 85%, 5 years after treatment. Thus, the period of service of a denture was unexpectedly long. Clinical studies show a great deal of loss of function 5 years after insertion, which did not correlate with patient satisfaction (reduced to 70–80%).

References

[1] Maryniuk, G. A., Kaplan, S. H. Longevity of restorations, survey results of dentist's estimates and attitudes. J Am Dent Assoc 1986; 112: 39–45.

[2] Maryniuk, G. A. In search of treatment longevity – a 30-year perspective. J Am Dent Assoc 1984; 109: 739–744.

[3] Leempoel, P. J. B., van't Hof, M. A., De Haan, A. F. J. Survival studies of dental restorations: criteria, methods and analysis. J Oral Rehabil 1989; 16: 387–394.

[4] Leempoel, P. J. B., Eschen, S., De Haan, A. F., van't Hof, M. A. An evaluation of crowns and bridges in a general dental practice. J Oral Rehabil 1985; 12: 515–528.

[5] Leempoel, P. J. B. Levensduur en nabehandelingen van kronen en conventionele bruggen in de algemene praktijk (Thesis). K. U. Nijmegen, 1987.

[6] Kerschbaum, Th., Paszyna, Ch., Klapp, S., Meyer G. Verweilzeit- und Risikofaktorenanalyse von festsitzendem Zahnersatz. Dtsch Zahnärztl Z 1991; 46: 20–24.

[7] Erpenstein, H., Kerschbaum, Th., Fischbach, H. Verweildauer und klinische Befunde bei Kronen und Brücken – eine Langzeitstudie. Dtsch Zahnärztl Z 1992; 47: 315–319.

[8] Kaplan, E. L., Meier, P. Nonparametric estimation from incomplete observations. J Am Stat Assoc 1958; 53: 457–481.

[9] Schwartz, N. L., Whitsett, L. D., Berry, Th. G., Stewart, J. L. Unserviceable crowns and fixed partial dentures: life-span and causes for loss of serviceability. J Am Dent Assoc 1970; 81: 1395–1491.

[10] Kerschbaum, Th., Thie, B. M. Funktionsverlust von festsitzendem Zahnersatz. Dtsch Zahnärztl Z 1986; 41: 2–7.

[11] Karlsson, S. Failures and length of service in fixed prosthodontics after long-term function. Swed Dent J 1989; 13: 185–192.

[12] Kerschbaum, Th., Leempoel, P. Kronen und Brücken. In: R. Voß/H. Meiners (ed.). Fortschritte der zahnärztlichen Prothetik und Werkstoffkunde. Vol. IV. pp. 109–136. München: Hanser, 1989.

[13] Kerschbaum, Th. Langzeitergebnisse und Konsequenzen. In: Hupfauf, L. (ed.). München: Urban & Schwarzenberg, 1988.

[14] Vermeulen, A. H. B. M. Een decennium evaluatie van partiële prothesen (Thesis). Nijmegen, 1984.

[15] Bergman, B., Hugosson, A., Olsson, C. O. Caries, periodontal status and prosthetic findings in patients with removable partial dentures: A ten-year longitudinal study. J Prosthet Dent 1982; 48: 506–514.

[16] Katay, L. Intensivbetreuung von Patienten mit herausnehmbaren Teilprothesen. Dtsch Zahnärztl Z 1990; 45: 410–413.

[17] Eismann, H. Longitudinalstudie zur Effektivität gegossener Teilprothesen. Dtsch Zahnärztl Z 1991; 46: 455–460.

[18] Carlsson, G. E., Ragnarsson, N., Åstrand, P. Changes in height of the alveolar process in edentulous segments. A longitudinal clinical and radiographic study of full upper denture cases with residual lower anteriors. Odontologisc Tidskr 1967; 75: 193–208.

[19] Carlsson, G. E., Ragnarsson, N., Åstrand, P. Changes in height of the alveolar process in edentulous segments, part II. Svensk Tandlaek T 1969; 62: 125–136.

[20] Sassen, H. Die Entwicklung von Okklusion und Funktion im Zeitraum von zwei Jahren nach Eingliederung von Teilprothesen. Dtsch Zahnärztl Z 1989; 44: 806–808.

[21] Sassen, H. Funktionelle Parameter und Okklusion von Teilprothesen in Abhängigkeit von der Art der Verbindungselemente. Dtsch Zahnärztl Z 1990; 45: 576–578.

[22] Käyser, A. F. Gebitsfuncties bij de verkorte tandbogen (Thesis). K. U. Nijmegen, 1975.

[23] Battistuzzi, P. G. F. C. M. Het gemutilieerde gebit (Thesis). Nijmegen, 1982.

[24] Bergman, B. Periodontal reactions related to removable partial dentures: A literature review. J Prosthet Dent 1987; 58: 454–458.

[25] Zarb, G. A., Bergman, B., Clayton, J. A., MacKay, H. F. Prosthodontic treatment for partially edentulous patients. St. Louis: Mosby, 1978.

[26] Butz-Jörgensen, E., Fleming, I. A 5-year longitudinal study of cantilevered fixed partial dentures compared with removable partial dentures in a geriatric population. J Prosthet Dent 1990; 64: 42–47.

[27] *Mühlenbein, F.* Longitudinale Analyse der Versorgung mit herausnehmbarem Zahnersatz bei Versicherten einer privaten Krankenversicherung (1974–1982). (Thesis) Köln, 1986.

[28] *Jonkman, R. E. G., Plooij, J.* Wortels onder een Kunstgebit, behouden? (Thesis). Nijmegen, 1992.

[29] *Carlsson, G. E., Otterland, A., Wennström, A.* Patient factors in appreciation of complete dentures. J Prosthet Dent 1967; *17:* 322–328.

[30] *Bergman, B., Carlsson, G. E.* Clinical long-term study of complete denture wearers. Acta Odont Scand 1985; *53:* 56–61.

[31] *Dette, K.-E., Stawitz, F., Taege, F.* Untersuchungen über die Funktionsbedingungen totaler Prothesen anhand ausgewählter Kriterien. Zahn Mund Kieferheilk 1987; *75:* 137–142.

[32] *Dette, K.-E.* Die Funktionsbedingungen totaler Prothesen. Zahn Mund Kieferheilk 1988; *76:* 409–412.

[33] *Kotkin, H.* Diagnostic significance of denture complaints. J Prosthet Dent 1985; *53:* 73–77.

[34] *Dolder, E., Wirz, J.* Die Steg-Gelenk-Prothese. Ein Leitfaden für Zahnarzt und Zahntechniker. Berlin: Quintessenz, 1982.

Chapter 4

An outline of patient selection and optimum treatment procedures

D. Harris

The availability of a secure and predictable means of bone anchorage, as provided by osseointegrated implants, has given rise to a whole new range of treatment possibilities in oral rehabilitation. The technical aspects of both achieving and maintaining osseo-integration require careful attention to detail in planning, surgical placement and healing, subsequent prosthetic loading and long-term maintenance. However, it should never be forgotten that, in themselves, implants cannot be a treatment except in so far as they contribute to the successful prosthetic rehabilitation of the patient. Failure to fully appreciate this, and to incorporate it into treatment planning, can lead to disastrous results in which all implants are integrated and yet the patient remains totally dissatisfied. Patients are not interested in osseointegration; they are only interested in the final outcome.

Patients, especially those who are fully edentulous, usually have very high expectations of the procedure for the following reasons:

(1) Psychological devastation can occur following loss of teeth. Social activities and interpersonal relationships can be disrupted to a great extent, especially among younger patients following sudden and traumatic loss of teeth. Functional problems associated with loose dentures, speech difficulties, pain and discomfort when eating and associated poor aesthetics can be significant. The prospects and expectations of having these problems solved are significant and very personal to the patient, as these could substantially improve their quality of life[1].

(2) It is necessary to undergo one or two surgical interventions and complex prosthetic procedures over a period of many months. On occasion, the surgery may be extensive and involves some pain and discomfort.

(3) The financial commitment to the procedure may be high.

Successfully rehabilitated patients are not slow to show their appreciation, but they can become disillusioned and bitterly disappointed when the results are less than expected.

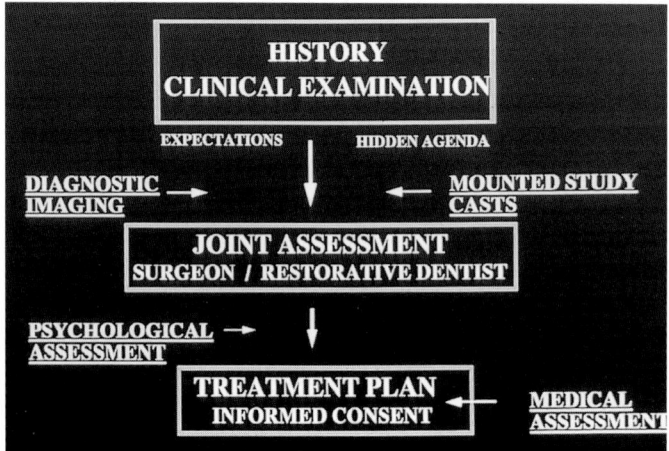

Fig. 1. Flow chart showing stages of treatment planning.

Reasons for patient dissatisfaction

Completed rehabilitation unsatisfactory

An inadequate clinical assessment can result in failure to place sufficient implants in an optimum position, or to allow the satisfactory construction of a fixed prosthesis when this has been promised. Failure to plan, visualize and predict the prosthetic result can result in speech problems, a bulky prosthesis, lack of tongue space, poor aesthetics and inability of a patient to maintain oral hygiene and health of adjacent soft tissues.

Unrealistic patient expectations

These may be caused by:

(1) Misunderstanding of a patient's psycho-logical needs and their reasons for undergoing treatment.

(2) Failure to communicate effectively and inform the patient as to what can and cannot be achieved.

(3) Psychological unsuitability of the patient.

No provision made for a contingency plan

The patient may not have been made aware of the possibility of more prolonged or modified treatment in the event of unforeseen difficulties arising, or as a result of an individual implant failure.

Treatment strategies

A fundamental prerequisite for the formulation of a successful treatment plan is the need for careful and detailed patient assessment and preparation. The surgeon and restorative dentist will need to collaborate closely to ensure that sufficient information is obtained to provide an acceptable treatment protocol. This protocol must be appropriate to the particular patient's needs, and should be sufficiently detailed for the individual to allow informed consent for the procedure to be carried out. The ultimate goal should be to provide a final rehabilitation for the patient in a way that will:

(1) Restore and maintain the health and function of all oral and associated tissues;
(2) Provide patient comfort (both physical and psychological);
(3) Provide a pleasing aesthetic result;
(4) Be within the capacity of the patient to maintain;
(5) Only necessitate treatment that is reasonable for the patient to undertake, with due regard to their medical status, age, physical capability and psychological capacity.

Initial interview and examination

The **primary** objective at the patient's initial interview and examination is to obtain a complete **history** and to carry out a careful **clinical examination**. A secondary objective is to gain an early impression of the patient's psychological make-up and an understanding of their motivation in seeking treatment. In particular, the patient's **expectations** concerning what they hope to achieve from the treatment should be discussed. It should be realized that patients may feel embarrassed or unsure about discussing some personal aspects of their problems and may well avoid stating the real reasons for attending. They should be encouraged to reveal any "**hidden agenda**", so that all expectations can be assessed. In all cases, the patient's **primary concern** or "**chief complaint**" must be identified and noted.

History

History taking is designed to provide an accurate profile of how the patient's quality of life is being affected by tooth loss, and by the consequent changes in associated tissues and in function. Only the patient can provide this information; it cannot be measured! It consists of three elements:

(1) Dental;
(2) Social/personal;
(3) Medical.

Dental

The dental aspects should include identification of all current problems from the patient's perspective. These may be categorized as follows:

(i) **Functional**: for example, unstable or loose dentures, inability to masticate efficiently, pain, TMJ disorders, difficulties with speech, gagging or ulceration and soreness of the mucosa;
(ii) **Psychological and Social**: for example, loss of self-esteem and confidence, feelings of guilt and insecurity, poor interpersonal relationships, social avoidance, lack of motivation and diminished libido;
(iii) **Aesthetic**: for example, loss of labial fullness and changes associated with a decrease in facial vertical dimension;
(iv) **Unrealistic**: for example, cannot accept ageing process, development of skin creases and lines not consequent upon tooth loss, dysmorphogenesis, paranoid delusions, psychological focus as a result of other life problems;

(v) **Not associated:** for example, xerostomia as a result of drug therapy or an underlying medical disorder such as Sjögrens syndrome, mucosal changes and "burning tongue" syndrome resulting from iron deficiency or *Candida* infection.

Social/personal

The impact and relevance of the dental condition to the patient's lifestyle should be explored, including possible limitations on social and sporting activities, and difficulties encountered at work. Wind instrument musicians, singers and actors may have particular problems. Special note should be made where speech, appearance and an absolute need for a fixed appliance are seen to be of special importance. Drinking and smoking habits should also be acertained.

Medical

A full and comprehensive review of a patient's medical history should be undertaken. If extensive surgery is necessary or a general anaesthetic is to be administered, it is advisable to have a full systems review carried out by a physician. In all cases, any condition that is likely to interfere with healing must be fully investigated e.g. diabetes, blood dyscrasias, irradiation of the bone or any condition associated with general disability or immunosuppression. Any medication currently being taken should be recorded, especially anticoagulants, steroids and antidepressants. A history of rheumatic fever, congenital or valvular heart disease or the presence of a prosthetic valve will necessitate appropriate antibiotic cover for any proposed surgery. All aller-

gies should be noted, especially to any antibiotics that may be prescribed[2, 3].

Clinical examination

A full examination of the stomatognathic system is carried out. This will include the soft tissues, bone, remaining teeth and associated tissues, as well as an extra-oral assessment.

The soft tissue and bone are examined for any sign of **underlying pathology,** e.g. premalignant conditions, candida, lichen planus, atrophic, hypertrophic, ulcerative, erosive or bullous conditions, cysts, swellings, sinuses, discharge or other signs of infection. Any oral manifestations of systemic disease should also be observed, e.g. mucosal changes as a result of anaemia or immunosuppression.

Inter-arch relationship and bone contours must be assessed. When treatment may include a removable prosthesis, careful note should be taken of any fraenal attachments, enlargement of bony or tuberosity areas, the presence of tori or any hyperplastic condition for which **preprosthetic surgery** might be considered necessary.

In partially dentate patients, a full **periodontal assessment** is made, as it is vitally important that any active periodontal infection is eliminated prior to implant placement and that, subsequently, a healthy periodontium is maintained[4].

All remaining **teeth** are examined to determine the condition of existing restorations and the presence of decay. In addition, a note should be made of any spacing, tilting or over-eruption. Inter-arch relationship is assessed. Any occlusal interferences in centric related closure, abnormalities in protrusive and lateral jaw movements, and any signs of parafunctional grinding habits should be recorded. **Temporomandibular** joint function must be examined with special reference to the presence of any "click" or deviation of the mandible on opening and closing movements. Palpation of the muscles of mastication, carried out when indicated. Mandibular opening must be adequate to allow access for proposed surgical and restorative procedures.

The extra-oral examination should include an assessment of facial symmetry, aesthetics, changes related to loss of vertical dimension, loss of labial support and whether the patient shows a "high lip-line". This latter finding will have important implications for aesthetics when replacing missing anterior teeth.

Expectations

At the first interview, an assessment should be made of the patient's knowledge and understanding of implant procedures and specific enquiries made as to what they hope to gain by undergoing the treatment. If they are dissatisfied with their present dental state, the source of this dissatisfaction needs to be carefully recorded. Educational and explanatory material appropriate to the problems can be provided as background information; in preparation for the next consultation.

Diagnostic imaging

This may include:
(1) Radiographs
   (i) Intra-oral periapical and bitewing views,
   (ii) Dental panoramic tomographs,
   (iii) Cephalometric views,
   (iv) Tomograms;
(2) CT imaging.

Radiographs are taken and examined with the following three objectives[5]. First, to ensure that there is a sufficient stock of well mineralized cortical and medullary bone to accommodate implants of adequate size in an optimum position for the prosthesis[6]. Secondly, to locate the position and proximity to potential implant sites of any adjacent anatomical structures that must not be damaged. These especially include the inferior dental and mental nerves, the maxillary antra and floor of nose, and adjacent teeth in partially dentate patients. Finally, to detect any bony abnormality or pathology that may interfere with implant placement. This will include the presence of impacted teeth, cysts, an enlarged incisive canal, retained amalgam fragments, evidence of periodontal disease or disorders of bone metabolism, e.g. Paget's disease or osteoporosis.

For a totally edentulous patient; a dental panoramic tomograph will clearly show the vertical height of the remaining alveolar and basal bone, the floor of the maxillary sinus and nasal apertures, the course of the inferior dental nerve and position of the mental foramen. Due to the variable magnitudes of enlargement which can differ, not only between machines but even within the one radiograph, exact measurements may be difficult. Bone density, distribution of cortical and medullary bone and evidence of localized abnormalities or pathology are usually well displayed. A cephalometric view is also required, to allow additional estimation of bone morphology and density and the maxilla/mandibular relationship. Partially dentate cases will need intra-oral periapical views to reveal greater detail concerning the teeth and bone at potential implant sites.

CT, scans and tomograms can provide essential additional information and meas-

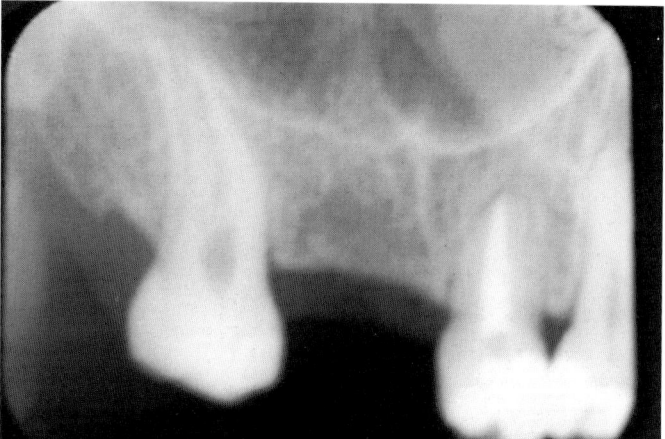

Fig. 2a

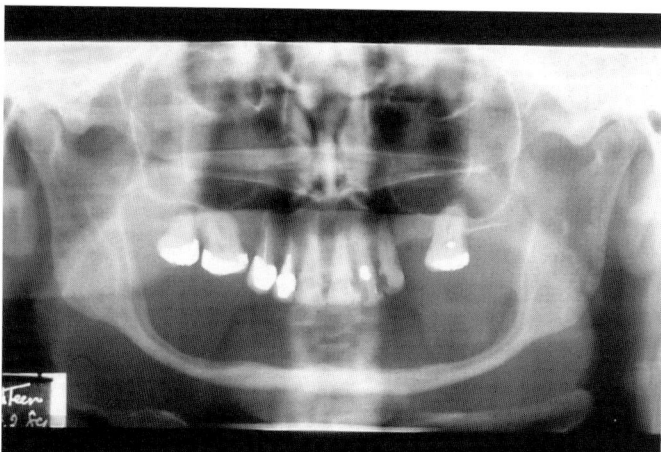

Fig. 2b

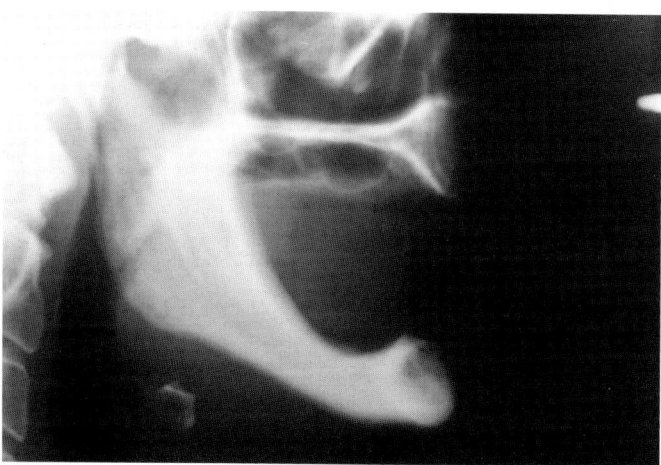

Fig. 2c

Fig. 2d

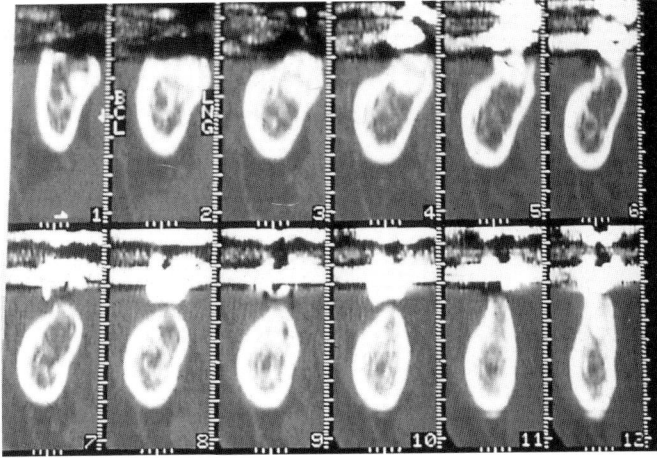

Fig. 2e

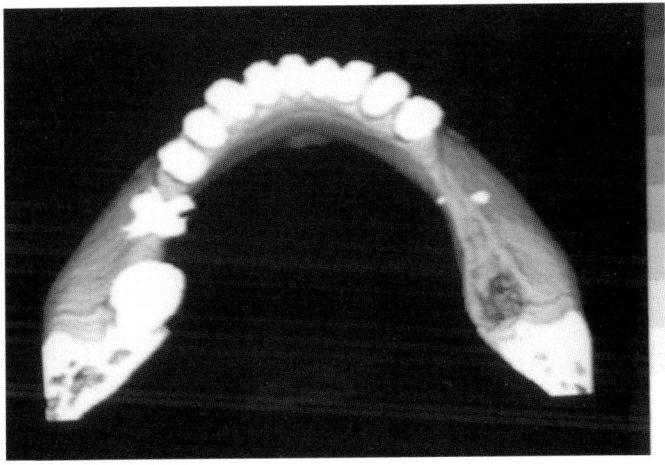

Fig. 2f

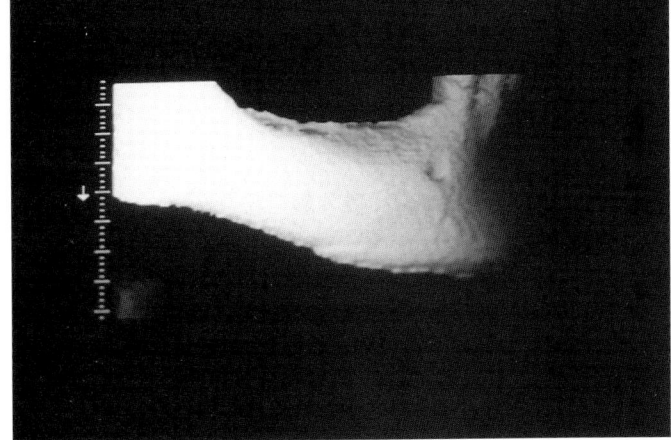

Fig. 2. Diagnostic imaging may include: intra-oral, periapical views (a), dental panoramic tomographs (b), cephalometric views (c), besides C.T, scan images and tomograms (d–f).

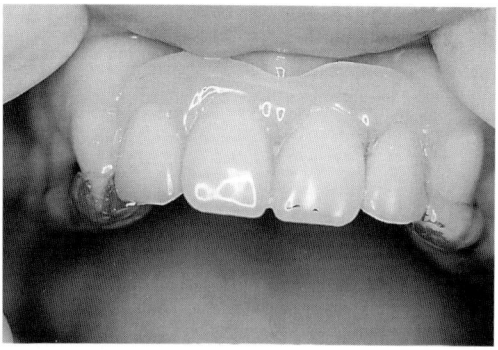

Fig. 3a

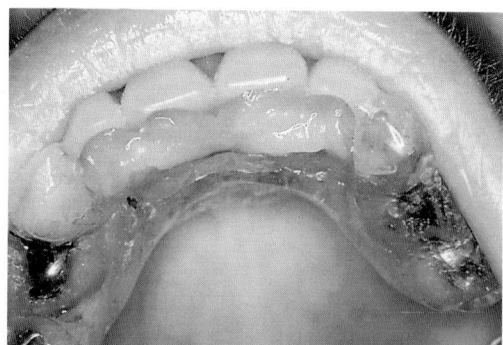

Fig. 3b

Fig. 3c

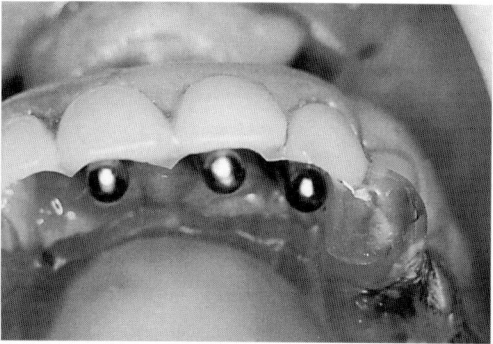

Fig. 3. Surgical templates improve the location and direction of the implants, resulting in optimal loading, aesthetics and phonetics. Before (a and b) and after (c) implant installation in the maxillary anterior area.

urements not available from standard radiographs. The indications are listed below[7, 8]:

(1) To assess the shape, quantity and mineralization of the mandibular bone above the inferior dental canal;
(2) To assess the shape, quantity and mineralization of maxillary bone available in relation to the maxillary antra and nasal floor.

Mounted study casts are an essential requirement for treatment planning in all clinical situations, even in totally edentulous patients. Examination of these models will help detect any difficulties that can arise from the presence of an unfavourable inter-arch relationship, e.g. a retruded maxilla or a prognathic mandible, cross-arch situations or lack of inter-arch space. Implant placement that ignores these latter conditions may preclude the eventual construction of a satisfactory prosthesis. In cases of partial edentulism, mounted models will also allow tooth position and interdental space available for implant placement to be accurately measured. Overeruption of teeth or an unfavourable occlusal plane may also be seen. The need for any preprosthetic surgery can also be studied and, where indicated, a diagnostic wax try-in and a **surgical guide or template**, to indicate optimum implant position, can be fabricated[9].

Where anterior teeth are being replaced, or aesthetics are of special importance, a diagnostic try-in for patient approval prior to treatment is essential.

Team assessment and treatment planning

In order to prepare an optimum treatment plan the above information must be jointly reviewed by both the restorative dentist and the surgeon. Based on the findings, it is the **prosthodontist's responsibility to provide a prosthetic prescription** that will fulfil the patient's needs with regard to health, function and aesthetics. It will also be necessary to indicate clearly where implants should be placed in order to achieve this. It is the **surgeon's responsibility to evaluate this prescription**, in the light of the clinical and radiographic assessment, and to **indicate the extent to which an adequate number of implants can be placed in an optimum position**. The following information should be readily available:

(1) Mounted study casts;
(2) Diagnostic wax-up and surgical template where indicated;
(3) Results from diagnostic imaging.

In drawing up a treatment strategy to present to the patient, the following considerations are of prime importance:

(1) The proposed treatment plan should address all aspects of the patient's present dissatisfaction with dental condition;
(2) The surgical procedures should be those which involve a **predictable prognosis based on substantial published evidence of recorded scientific data;**[10]
(3) The procedures involved must be within the patient's mental and physical abilities to undergo;

(4) The procedures should not cause the patient any harm, e.g. sensory nerve damage or, in the event of failure, cause a deterioration in the dental condition, e.g. excessive bone loss. *Primum non nocere* (first do no harm).

In considering sites for implant placement, it is important to evaluate whether the bone topography will allow them to be placed in an optimum position, particularly if fixed restorations are planned in the maxilla. Implants placed too far lingually, or buccally, or emerging in an interdental space, can greatly compromise the prosthetic result. Implant placement in the posterior mandibular area may not be possible owing to an inadequate volume of bone above the inferior dental nerve, or in the maxilla owing to insufficient bone beneath the maxillary antra or nasal floor. A number of supplementary procedures are available that may help to overcome these anatomical limitations. These include **bone augmentation** by means of **guided tissue regeneration** techniques, **bone grafting procedures** and **nerve transposition. In each individual case, careful consideration should be given to the possibility and advisability of such treatments and the implications for achieving a predictable prognosis**[11, 12].

In some clinical situations it may be found that an optimum prosthetic rehabilitation cannot be fully achieved, or that the end result is not fully predictable. Any shortcomings must be carefully evaluated in the context of the patient's expectations. Before discussing the proposed treatment with the patient, consideration should be given as to whether further investigations are indicated.

Informed consent

Before consenting to undergo the proposed treatment, the patient must understand and be made fully aware of all aspects of the treatment, especially with regard to any potential **benefits** and **risks**[13]. They must also be given clear information on **alternative treatments** (see chapter 2) for their condition, and this includes the possibility of having **no treatment at all**.

They should be left in no doubt as to the final prosthetic result that is likely to be achieved, how long it is estimated that the total prosthetic and surgical treatment will take, and how much it will cost. **Where anterior maxillary teeth are to be replaced, they should see and agree with the aesthetics on a wax "try-in".**

If the provision of a fixed prosthesis is a high priority, or is the only reason for undertaking treatment, it must be made clear whether there are any possibilities of this not being achieved in the event of a fixture failure. In all cases; a contingency plan should be discussed, which may include the possibility of implant failure, further surgery, provision of a removable or a temporary prosthesis, prolonged treatment and grafting or augmentation of bone.

In all cases the team must be satisfied that the patient really understands and appreciates the limits to what can be achieved, is aware of and accepts any possible shortcomings in the expected end result and knows what is required to ensure long-term maintenance of implants and prostheses[14]. Optimum treatment requires that only the minimal amount of intervention be undertaken to correct the patient's problems. On occasion, placing fewer implants to support a removable prosthesis, thus allowing a patient to easily maintain the health of the peri-implant tissues, and still solve their functional problems, might prove to be most appropriate.

The patient should be informed of the expected post-operative course of any surgical procedure and any possible side-effects that may be encountered. There is no universal rule with regard to this and it must clearly be related to the type and extent of surgery, as well as to the presence of adjacent anatomical structures. In addition, different countries have varying requirements and medicolegal precedents that will influence the extent of detail that is required. However, such information may well need to include the possibility of altered or loss of sensation in the mental region or upper lip, fracture of the jaw, penetration of the floor of the sinus or nose, swelling, bruising, haemorrhage, infection or damage to adjacent teeth. They should also be informed of any periods when they will need to be without teeth replacements. Consideration may be given to staging the various procedures so that an intermediate prosthesis can be provided; to avoid the need to wear a removable prosthesis at any stage.

It should be decided, in consultation with the patient, whether the surgical treatment is best carried out on an in-patient basis or as a day-stay procedure. Consideration should also be given to whether the extent of the surgery, or the physical or psychological capacities of the patient, indicate that the procedure should be undertaken with either:

(1) Local analgesia alone;
(2) Local analgesia in conjunction with oral or intravenous sedation;[15]
(3) Under a general anaesthetic.

This decision will not always be influenced by clinical need alone, but may be dictated by the availability of facilities for sedation and anaesthesia in a particular country.

Nonetheless, everything possible should be done to ensure that the treatment will upset the patient as little as possible and to take into account the large numbers in the population who are extremely anxious when undergoing any treatment in the oral cavity. A definitive treatment plan may now be discussed with the patient. This may include preliminary preparatory procedures prior to implant placement, for example elimination of all active periodontal disease or other source of infection, preprosthetic surgery and treatment of any underlying pathology. Consideration may need to be given to tooth removal or orthodontic movement. The possibility of any **underlying medical disorders** that may influence the patient's ability to undergo treatment may necessitate referral to a **physician** for evaluation, especially if general anaesthesia is to be administered. Patients should be made aware that **smoking can adversely affect successful osseointegration**. On occasion, a **psychological assessment** may be advisable if the patient's responses or inability to appreciate the true nature of the proposed treatment are uncertain. **It is the experience of every team providing implant-based treatment that they have treated at least one patient who, in retrospect, they realize was psychologically unsuited to the procedure.**

Summary

Optimum treatment results will be obtained more frequently in a wide variety of clinical situations by adopting a team approach to implant-based reconstruction. An appropriate team consists of a surgeon and restorative dentist working in close collaboration. Additional team members include; a nurse hygienist and technician and, where necessary, a physician, an anaesthetist and a psychologist. A consistent and predictable outcome can be achieved only with good patient selection and the development of a successful treatment strategy for a patient who has been fully informed.

References

[1] *Blomberg, S.,* and *Lindqvist, L. W.* Psychological reactions to edentulousness and treatment with jawbone anchored bridges. Acta Psychiatr Scand 1983; *68:* 251.

[2] *Peterson, L. J.* Antibiotic prophylaxis against wound infection in oral and maxillofacial surgery. J Oral Maxillofac Surg 1990; *48:* 617–620.

[3] *Little, J. W.* Antibiotic prophylaxis for prevention of bacterial endocarditis and infectious major joint prostheses. Current Op Dent 1992; *2:* 93–101.

[4] *Quiryen, M.,* and *Listgarten, M. A.* The distribution of bacterial morphotypes around natural teeth and titanium implants ad modum Brånemark. Cli Oral Implant Res 1990; *1:* 8–12.

[5] *Hollender, L.* Radiographic examination of endosseous implants in the jaws. In: *Worthington, P.,* and *Brånemark, P.-I.* (eds), Advanced osseointegration surgery. pp. 80–93. Berlin: Quintessence Publ Co, 1992.

[6] *Mecall, R. A., Rosenfeld, A. L.* The influence of residual ridge resorptive patterns on implant fixture placement and tooth position. Part 1. Int J Periodont Restor Dent 1992; *11:* 8–23.

[7] *Quirynen, M., Lamoral, T., Dekeyser, C., Peene, P., van Steenberghe, D., Bonte, J.,* and *Baert, A.* The C.T. scan standard reconstruction for reliable jaw bone volume determination. Int J Oral Maxillofac Implants 1990; *5:* 384–389.

[8] *Smith, J. P., Borrow, J. W.* Reformatted C.T. imaging for implant planning. Oral Maxillofac Clin North Am 1991; *3:* 805–325.

[9] *Cowan, P.* Surgical templates for the placement of osseointegrated implants. Quintessence Int 1990; *21:* 391–396.

[10] *Albrektsson, T., Zarb, G. A., Worthington, P.,* and *Eriksson, A.* The long-term efficacy of currently used dental implants: A review and proposed criteria for success. Int J Oral Maxillofac Implants 1986; *1:* 11–22.

[11] *Wachtel, H. C., Langford, A., Bernimoulin, J-P., Reichart, P.* Guided bone regeneration next to osseointegrated implants in humans. Int J Oral Maxillofac Implants 1991; *6:* 127–135.

[12] *Adell, R., Lekholm, U., Grondahl, K., Brånemark, P.-I., Lindstrom, J.,* and *Jacobson, M.* Reconstruction of severely resorbed edentulous maxillae using osseointegrated fixtures in immediate autogenous bone grafts. Int J Oral Maxillofac Implants 1990; *5:* 223–246.

[13] *Harris D.* Osseointegrated implants. Annual Report: The Medical Protection Society (London) 1988; *96:* 47–48.

[14] *Ortan, G. S., Steele, D. I.,* and *Wolinsky, L. E.* The dental professional's role in monitoring and maintainance of tissue integrated prostheses. Int J Oral Maxillofac Implants, 1989; *4:* 305–310.

[15] *Harris, D., O'Boyle, C.,* and *Barry H.* Oral sedation with temazepam: controlled comparison of a soft gelatin capsule formulation with intravenous diazepam. Br Dent J 1987; *8:* 297–301.

Chapter 5
Part I

Biomaterials and interfaces

B. Kasemo and J. Lausmaa

Introduction

Let us begin by considering a foreign material, suddenly inserted into a tissue. Before insertion the tissue is undisturbed. The effect of the implantation is twofold: first, there is the tissue damage created by the surgical procedure; secondly, there is now a foreign body, presenting a foreign surface for the tissue to interact with. The important questions in this situation are: Will the material surface affect the healing process, and in what way? Will the biological system attack and attempt to modify the material and its surface and if so, how does this happen? We now know that different materials have different effects on the tissue response, and that different materials are required for various types of tissue, etc. Such knowledge originally evolved empirically. Materials that were thought likely to function well in the tissue (often as a result of experiences with non-biological applications) were tried out with varying degrees of success, until, eventually, it became clear which materials were acceptable and which were not. In the present chapter, we focus on the questions listed above, and specifically on those related to the material surface and how it will influence, and be influenced by, its biological host. For a more extensive treatment of the subject, the interested reader is referred to previous reviews and books on the subject.[1–3]

Material and surface properties

Selected properties of solid materials

The properties of materials (mechanical strength, density, electrical and thermal conductivity, hardness, reactivity/stability, etc) are to a great extent determined by the chemical composition of the material and the type of binding that keeps the constituent atoms together. In solids the atoms are densely arranged (typically circa 10^{23} atoms/cm^3, which corresponds to interatomic spacings of a few times 10^{-8} cm) and are relatively fixed in their positions. The atoms in solids are often arranged in regular patterns; this is called the crystal structure. Adjacent atoms are bound to each other by chemical bonds (metallic bonding, covalent or ionic bonding, etc), formed by the valence electrons of the constituent atoms. In real materials the regular pattern of atoms often extends over only circa 1 μm, sometimes less and sometimes more. Each unit, with its regular atomic arrangement, is called a crystallite or crystalline grain. The crystallites are stacked together, with the boundaries, the so-called grain boundaries, where the atomic arrangement is less regular. Such materials are said to be polycrystalline. In exceptional cases, the whole material is a single crystal. This is the case, for example, with gem stones.

The mechanical properties of a particular material, such as strength, ductility, brittleness, etc, are a complex function of the local chemical composition and bonding between adjacent atoms, the grain structure, the concentration of defects and irregularities other than at the grain boundaries (eg dislocations and vacancies), and the presence of additives and impurities in the material. These factors can, to a large extent, be varied by the material processing, and are therefore used to produce quite different properties in a single type of material.

Surface properties

In order to describe some properties of surfaces it is appropriate to start by considering a solid under vacuum. By breaking the solid into two pieces, two new surfaces are created. The surface consists of the outermost atomic layer of the solid and thus constitutes a termination of the extended, three-dimensional lattice. The breaking of the bonds in the solid results in a thermodynamically unstable (energetically unfavourable) situation, since it increases the total energy of the system. This increase in energy is often called the surface energy. Microscopically, the surface energy is the result of the unsaturated (dangling) bonds which occur when the bonds in the solid are

broken. In vacuum, the surface energy can be lowered by rearrangement (relaxation) of the surface atomic positions, or by a reconstruction of the surface which lowers the number of unsaturated bonds.

The chemical composition of surfaces often differs from that of the corresponding bulk (unless, of course, the material is composed of a single element). For compound materials it may be thermodynamically favourable if one element is more common at the surface than the others. Low-concentration impurities from the bulk may diffuse to the surface in a process called segregation. In alloys, one or more of the alloy constituents are often found in greater concentrations at the surface. This is the case, for example, for stainless steel and for the Ti6A14V alloy, which have higher concentrations of Cr and Al, respectively, at their surfaces. Surfaces may also contain chemical impurities. These can exist as single atoms/molecules or adsorbed overlayers. The latter type of surface contamination is further discussed below.

Most of the microstructural features outlined previously also apply to surfaces. Surfaces can be single-crystalline, polycrystalline or amorphous. They also exhibit topography and roughness at different scales of dimension (from atomic level up to circa 1–100 μm), which will be strongly influenced by the way the surface is prepared. Another major factor which influences surface properties is their interaction with the environments they are exposed to, which will be discussed below.

Interactions at surfaces

A fresh surface placed in an environment is, as mentioned above, thermodynamically unstable. The environment may be a gas, a liquid, or a complex biological system, and

Fig. 1. The interaction potential, U(r), as a function of distance from surface, for a particle approaching a surface. The shaded curve shows the derivative of U(r) with respect to r, ie the force F(r) experienced by the particle. At distances greater than a few nm there is no interaction between the surface and the particle. At smaller distances (≤ 1 nm) the potential decreases rapidly, and the particle is subject to an attraction force. The potential goes through a minimum, typically a few tenths of nm from the surface, and increases rapidly at even smaller distances. At the potential minimum, the attraction and repulsion forces cancel out, and the particle thus becomes trapped at the surface (adsorbed). The dashed curve illustrates the case where there is a potential barrier for adsorption.

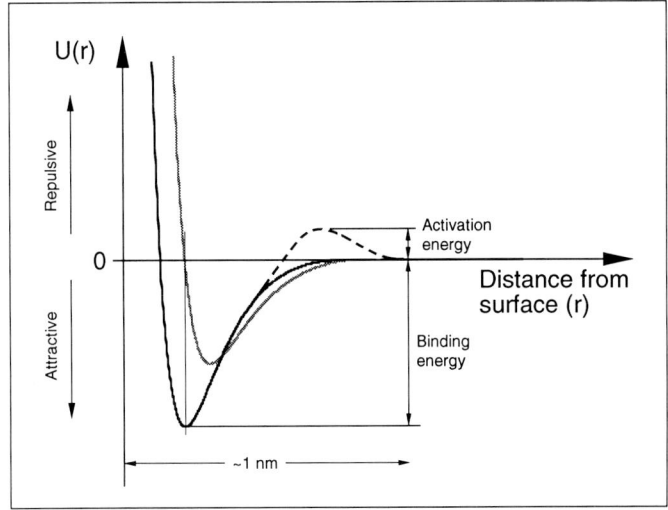

it is inevitable that the surface will come into close contact with its molecular constituents. The events that will occur are determined by the interaction potential between the surface and the environment. For simplicity, let us choose a gaseous environment. A typical interaction potential U(r) as a function of the distance, r, between a gas molecule and a surface, is shown by the solid line in Fig. 1. In a classical sense, U(r) represents the potential energy of the combined molecule-surface system at different distances, r, between them. The shaded line represents the derivative of U(r), $dU/dr = -F(r)$, which is the force exerted by the surface on the gas particle. At large distances, (> few nm) there is virtually no (direct) interaction between the particle and the surface. Closer to the surface, the potential energy decreases rapidly with distance; in other words, the particle experiences an attracting force. The potential goes through a minimum, where the force is zero, typically at a few Ångströms (10^{-10} m) from the sur-

face. Even closer, the interaction potential increases sharply and the particle is thus subjected to a strong repulsive force. This is a very common phenomenon: an attracting force – a minimum – and a repulsive force at close distance.

The surface–particle system will therefore have its lowest energy at the distance where the potential minimum occurs. Here, the attraction and repulsion forces cancel out, and the gas molecule will become bound (adsorbed) to the surface. The gas molecule may also break into fragments (dissociate) upon adsorption, but for this to occur there may be an activation barrier in the potential curve (dashed line in Fig. 1). Depending on the depth of the potential minimum, the particle can be irreversibly or reversibly bound to the surface. In the latter case, the particle will return to the gas phase. This process is called desorption.

The detailed shape of the interaction potential (and thus the chemical properties of the

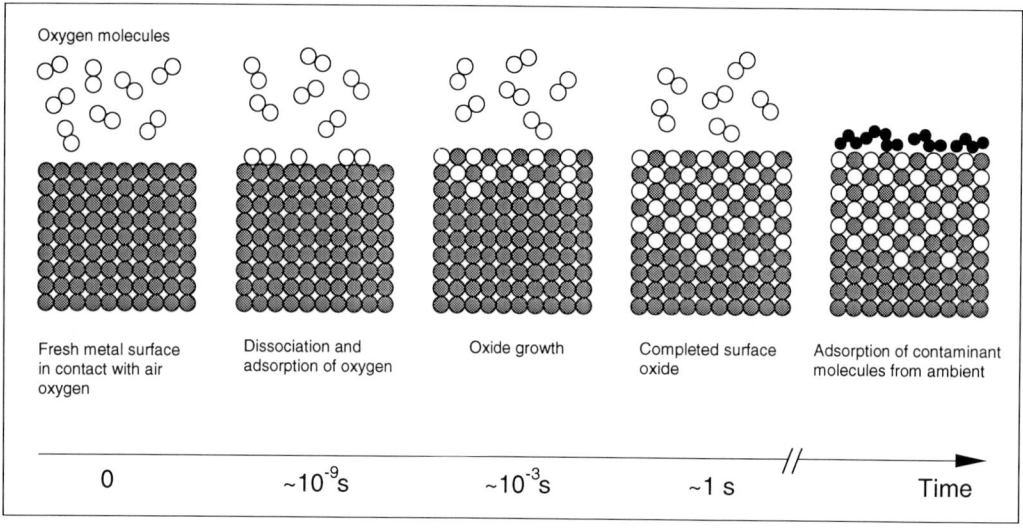

Fig. 2. Schematic illustration of the formation of an oxide overlayer on a freshly created metal surface. The illustration on the right shows the formation of an adsorbed contamination layer over the surface oxide.

surface) will be determined by the local properties of the surface (electronic structure, microstructure and defects, chemical composition, etc), as well as by the properties of the interacting particles in, for example; the liquid.

In a reactive environment, such as air or water, the unsaturated surface bonds will quickly (< 1 second) react to form new bonds and compounds (Fig. 2), thus lowering the surface energy. Well-known examples include the oxide overlayers which form on almost all metals (except the noble metals), and hydroxylated ceramic surfaces, respectively. Oxidation proceeds via dissociation of oxygen molecules and oxygen (and/or metal) ion diffusion from (and/or to) the metal–environment interface. In most metals, the thermodynamic driving force to form oxides is very strong. For kinetic reasons (usually transport limitation), the oxidation process is virtually complete at fairly low oxide thicknesses (a

few nanometers). Even after such surface reactions have occurred, the surface still tends to lower its surface energy, for example by binding molecules from the air, leading to surface contamination. For this reason, most surfaces are covered by a monolayer of adsorbed contaminant molecules (often hydrocarbons).

Before going on to discuss interactions at the material–tissue interface, some important points to remember are summarized below:

(1) The creation of a surface involves the formation of unsaturated surface bonds that tend to react with the environment, and so lower the surface energy.

(2) Surfaces frequently have a different chemical composition and microstructure, compared to the corresponding bulk material.

(3) Most surfaces are heterogeneous, ie their composition, microstructure and

surface structure (roughness and topography) show variations accross the surface.

(4) Surfaces continuously interact with the environment, by adsorbing molecules, and by chemical reactions with adsorbed molecules. The direct interaction takes place at a distance ≤ 1 nm from the surface.

(5) The properties of surfaces are strongly influenced by the way they are prepared.

Example: titanium implant surfaces

The surface properties of titanium are, to a large extent, determined by the surface oxide, which almost always covers the metal. The characteristics of titanium implant surfaces are now quite well known, thanks to a large number of studies using electron spectroscopic and microscopic methods[2, 4-8]. These and other studies have provided extensive evidence that the surface properties of different Ti implants are a function of the history of the implant. The conditions during oxidation (temperature, type and concentration of oxiding species, presence of contaminants, etc), strongly influence the physical and chemical properties of the oxide layer. The initial surface oxide (formed, for example, during machining) is frequently modified during later stages of the preparation of an implant and in most cases will be covered by a hydrocarbon contamination layer, typically one monolayer of molecules or less in thickness, under clean conditions.

Properties and processes at the interface

Properties at the interface

From the discussion in the previous section it follows that, owing to the short range of the physical and chemical forces involved, direct interactions between a material and the environment take place in a very narrow region, close to the surface. The direct interaction between the biomaterial and the tissue takes place in a zone which extends, at most, a few nanometers into the biological system. Thus, the surface properties of biomaterials are a determining factor for these interactions. This does not mean that the bulk of the biomaterial and the biosystem are irrelevant. Important secondary reactions, and indirect interactions can take place in both these regions.

Before discussing the processes which are likely to occur at the interface, we will first identify some of the protagonists and the size ranges at which they appear (Fig. 3). The dimensions of interest cover a very wide range, from the macroscopic level (circa 1–10 mm) down to the microscopic (molecular and atomic) level (circa 0.1–1 nm).

Biological components

Among the biological components, the smallest structures are the water molecules and the (mostly hydrated) ions of the physiological fluid. Commonly occurring ionic species include, for example, Na^+, Cl^-, Mg^{2+}, Ca^{2+}, and PO^{3-}_4. On a somewhat larger scale, there are the building blocks of the proteins, the amino acids. The amino acids are bound together in specific sequences to form long chains, peptides,

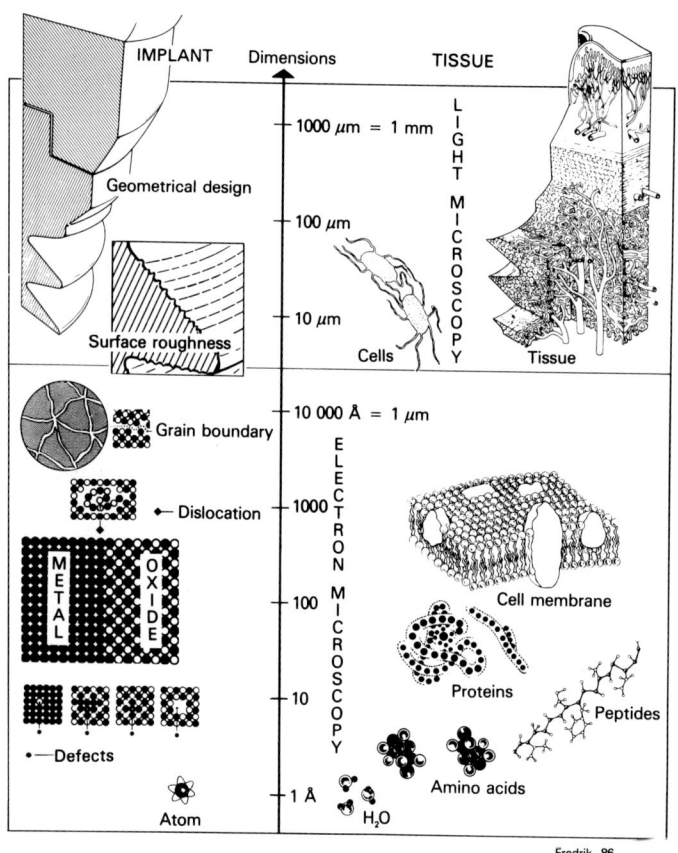

Fig. 3. Schematic illustration of the approximate dimensions of some typical structures found at the interface between tissue and implant (in this case a Ti dental implant). Note that within each size range, structures of corresponding dimensions can be found on each side of the interface.

Fredrik -86
© P-I Brånemark
Kasemo & Lausmaa

which form the backbone of the proteins. The proteins belong to a large class of complex biomolecules, typically circa 1–10 nm in size, and are characterized by various unique and dynamic structures which determine their multitude of biological functions. Different proteins play important roles in a number of vital functions, for example, in the transport of oxygen (by haemoglobin) between the lungs and the cells, in the coagulation of blood (e.g. fibrin and fibrinogen), and in the catalysis of biochemical reactions (enzymes). In the same size range as the proteins, there are also other biological macromolecules, such as lipids and carbohydrates.

Further up the dimensional scale, even more complex biological structures are found, including the cell membranes which form the surfaces of cells. Cell membranes are composed of a double layer of lipids, arranged so that their hydrophilic ends are facing out from the bilayer. They also contain a variety of mobile, functional groups and proteins. Finally, at the 1–10 μm level, we find various types of cells, which determine the macroscopic organization and behaviour of the host tissue. At this level, bacteria, which may be present at the interface, are also found.

The biomaterial surface

Among the inorganic components of the interface, the smallest structures of interest are the atoms (or ions or molecules) and their geometrical arrangement (crystal structure) at the biomaterial surface. At this level, one also finds various atomic defects (vacancies, interstitials and impurities) and grain boundaries (see above). Typical dimensions for surface oxide and contamination layer thicknesses, and dislocations are roughly 1 nm to 100 nm. On a larger scale (1–100 μm) the surface is characterized by the grain structure. Finally, at the macroscopic level, geometric shape and design of the implant lie in the region of about 1–10 mm. The surface topographic features can vary over the same size range. Steps may be one to many atomic diameters high, and ridges, grooves, pits, etc, may be of any size from atomic to macroscopic dimensions. Most of the structures mentioned above can be expected to significantly influence the function of the biomaterial, even if there is no change in average surface chemical composition. However, the chemical composition of the surface is the more important factor of the two in determining the adsorption properties and chemical reactivity of the surface. The fact that structures of different types occur in all the abovementioned size ranges, both in the biological system and on the surface, leads to the following general statement. A structure on the surface can always be created to match a biological component in shape and size. For proteins, such structures would be circa 1 nm in size, while for cells they would be on the 1–10 μm scale. It is very likely that such microstructures will combine through purely chemical interaction to produce synergistic structure-chemistry derived interactions at all relevant size levels.

Molecular processes at the interface

This section will identify some of the molecular processes that are likely to occur at implant–tissue interfaces. The behaviour and function of different cells, and the influence of bacteria, at the interface will not be covered here. (The interested reader is referred to reviews on the subject in Davies[3]. Most of the examples referred to involve Ti, but many of the concepts which are presented are equally applicable to other materials.

Ion release and surface remodelling

Most biomaterials are not inert in physiological environments, but undergo some corrosion or degradation. It is well known that metal implants can give rise to elevated metal ion concentrations; both locally and systemically[9]. Related phenomena may occur with polymer materials, which can degrade in the physiological environment by releasing monomers or additives. (This can be used to advantage in drug administration devices and sutures). Another biomaterial, hydroxyapatite, also interacts actively with the biological system, and these complex chemical reactions eventually lead to an apparent chemical bond with bone.

Titanium is known to be highly resistant to corrosion in aqueous and saline solutions. However, observations from both *in vitro* and *in vivo* experiments show that Ti surfaces may undergo significant changes in

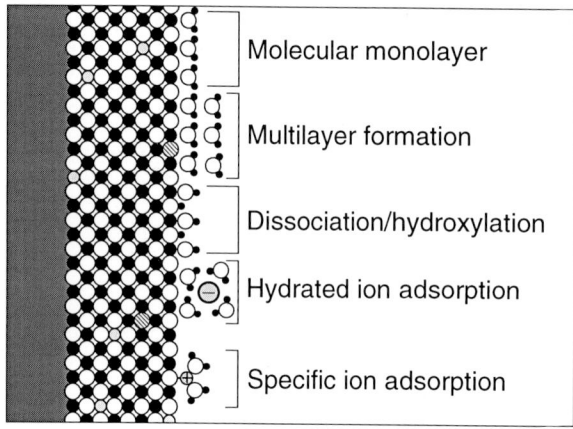

Molecular monolayer

Multilayer formation

Dissociation/hydroxylation

Hydrated ion adsorption

Specific ion adsorption

Fig. 4. Schematic illustration of possible interactions between water and ions at surfaces.

the biological milieu, over periods extending from a few seconds, up to several years. Examples of inorganic reactions at Ti surfaces which may be relevant to the *in vitro* situation are briefly considered below.

Sundgren et al.[10] analysed surface layers on Ti implants which had been implanted in humans for periods of up to 10 years or more. On those implants which had been in place for the longest period, the oxide thickness had grown from the original 5 nm to over 200 nm. In addition, increased levels of Ca and P were observed in the surface layers, indicating that ions from the physiological environment had become incorporated in the oxide on the implants.

In vitro studies have demonstrated measurable ion release rates for Ti and Ti6A14V exposed to various model physiological solutions[11, 12]. Typical Ti, Al and V ion concentrations detected in the model solutions after 3–4 months of exposure are in the range 0.1–1 ppm per cm^2 of sample area. With time there is an increase in oxide layer, leading to a decrease in the ion release rate. Although; as yet, no adverse effects of Ti dissolution *in vivo* have been observed; the very long-term effects of such dissolution are still unknown. *Tengvall* et al.[13] have shown that Ti surfaces exposed to hydrogen peroxide solutions react to form a complex gel, composed of titanium peroxyhydroxides. This is an interesting observation, since, during inflammation, H_2O_2 is produced by activated cells; this means that a Ti-gel may form at Ti implant surfaces. Other interesting *in vitro* observations have been reported by *Hanawa* et al.[14]. They immersed different metal samples in a physiological solution and analysed the surface films formed after different exposure times. Ca and P deposition was detected at the surfaces of most of the investigated metals, and the effect was more pronounced on Ti than on other materials. The chemical states of the Ca and P were also found to be almost identical to those in hydroxyapatite, the mineral constituent of bone.

Water–surface interaction

Very little is actually known about the microscopic interactions between the surface and the biological components at real implant–tissue interfaces, but it is possible

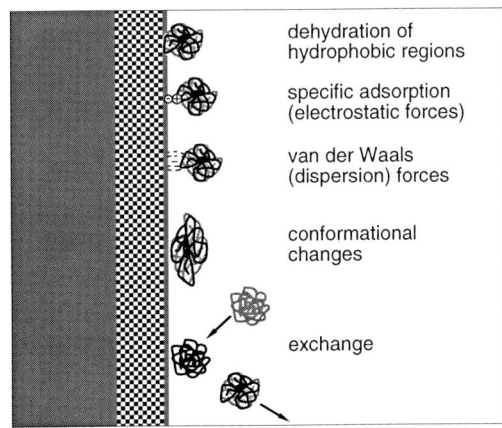

dehydration of
hydrophobic regions

specific adsorption
(electrostatic forces)

van der Waals
(dispersion) forces

conformational
changes

exchange

Fig. 5. Schematic illustration of different ways in which proteins may bind to surfaces. The lower part of the picture illustrates an exchange reaction.

to postulate the following series of events. Contact with the physiological fluid initially leads to water adsorption at the implant surface, which occurs very quickly (circa 10^{-6}–10^{-8} seconds). Some of the water molecules bind weakly to the surface, while others are more strongly bound (chemisorbed), or even dissociate to form hydroxyl (OH-) groups at the surface, leading to hydroxylation of the surface. Different water–surface interactions are schematically illustrated in Fig. 4. It has been clearly established that various surfaces interact differently with water molecules[15]. The different degrees of hydrophilicity or hydrophobicity exhibited in the water–surface interaction, are a macroscopic manifestation of such differences at the molecular level.

Various ionic species (Na$^+$, Ca^{2+}, Cl$^-$, phosphates, etc) are also present at the surface and in the hydration layer. They may become indirectly and weakly bound to the surface via their hydration (water) shells (Fig. 4). Alternatively, they may bind more strongly and form direct bonds to surface atoms (ions) by shedding their hydration shells.

The surface layer of an implant *in vivo* is therefore initially covered by a hydration layer consisting of water molecules, hydroxyl groups and ions, and this changes with time. The composition and structure of the hydration layer is expected to vary considerably for different surfaces. Different types of inorganic reactions may take place at different times after implantation, as pH, ion concentrations, and so on, change. After the initial formation of the hydration layer, various types of biomolecules will appear at, and interact with, the (hydrated) surface.

Biomolecule adsorption

The majority of proteins (and other biomolecules) arrive at the surface at a later stage than the water and the ions, since they are larger, have lower diffusion rates, and lower concentrations in the physiological liquid. Several possibilities for biomolecule binding to the surface can be postulated (Fig. 5). One important mechanism for protein adsorption to (hydrophobic) surfaces is dehydration of the hydrophobic regions on the surface and protein, respectively. This type

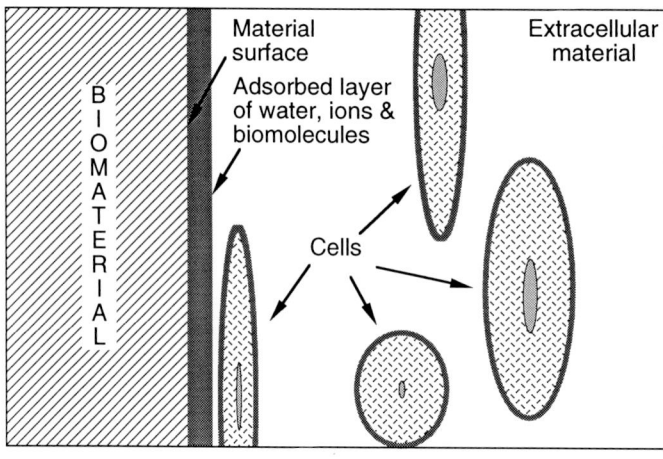

Fig. 6. A simplified representation of an interface. The cells interact with the surface via the adsorbed (and dynamic) layer of water, ions and biomolecules. The surface properties of the biomaterial, which may change significantly with time *in vivo*, constitute an important starting point for the development of the interface, since they govern the interaction with water, ions, and biomolecules.

of interaction is often referred to as hydrophobic interaction. Other possible binding mechanisms are weak adsorption by *van der Waals* (dispersion) forces or by hydrogen bonding, by dipole interactions, or stronger adsorption by ionic or covalent bonds.

There is a large body of experimental evidence concerning biomolecule adsorption phenomena at different surfaces, particularly for proteins[16, 17], which can be expected to act at the interface between implant and tissue. It is often observed that high-energy (hydrophilic) surfaces adsorb less proteins than low-energy (hydrophobic) surfaces, although protein-specific exceptions exist. Other surface properties, such as surface charge, polarity, and mobility, are also important factors for determining how specific proteins adsorb to surfaces. Protein adsorption may be either reversible or irreversible, and most often only one monolayer or less is adsorbed. Proteins may undergo conformational (structural) changes in the adsorption process at some surfaces. Such conformational changes may change the function of proteins, which could have biological con-

sequences. One type of process which is probably of particular significance in the *in vivo* situation is exchange (Fig. 5), i.e. the replacement of weakly bound proteins by others which bind more strongly (the Vroman effect).

Relation to cellular activity

One important consequence of the molecular interactions between the implant and biomolecules, outlined above, is that *in vivo* the surface will inevitably become covered by water, ions and biomolecules. It is with this dynamic hydration and biomolecule coating that the surrounding cells and tissue will interact (Fig. 6).

The cells may interact with the surface via molecular groups in or on their membranes and via the various biochemical signal substances they express and ingest. The types of cells which will proliferate at the interface, and change their behaviour; are likely to be influenced by, the composition and organization of the adsorbed biomolecule layer. Depending on the properties of the original surface, as well as on the type and state of the host tissue, healing-in conditions, etc, healing-in conditions, etc, the complex interplay at the interface may or may not lead to the successful co-existence of tissue and implant. Identification of the organic and inorganic components present at the interface, and an understanding of their functions and roles in the macroscopic development of the interface, constitute one of the most important challenges involved in understanding and controlling biomaterial–tissue interactions today.

The role of specific surface properties for tissue response and clinical function

There is ample experimental evidence in the literature to show that biomaterials with different chemical compositions trigger different biological responses. The influence of low levels of impurities, alloys, or surface contaminants, however, has not yet been studied systematically. For example, the effects of molecular surface contamination layers on the function of implants is not known. Nevertheless, it is important to realize that the contamination layer is there, and that its extent and exact composition vary considerably, depending both on the original material and on its preparation.
The influence of surface roughness and topography on the behaviour of tissues and cells has been studied extensively. Surface roughness and porosity at the level of circa 100 μm and larger has been shown to result in tissue ingrowth. It is also clear that surface structural features roughly in the 1–10 μm range directly influence the behaviour of individual cells, both *in vitro* and *in vivo*. This has, for example, been shown by *Brunette* et al.[18], who used microfabricated surfaces to systematically study the influence of surface structures of different

size and shape on the behaviour of endothelial cells, fibroblasts and osteoblasts. The < 1 μm range has been less well studied, but there are reasons to expect that structural features also within this range can influence the biological response, via interactions with cellular components and biomolecules of corresponding dimensions, such as cell processes, molecular groups expressed at the cell membrane, and proteins or other biomolecules. From a functional point of view, there are probably optimal levels of surface roughness for different applications. However, it is currently not possible to predict in which size ranges these optima occur. It is also important to point out that surface composition, microstructure and topography are likely to influence the biological response in a concerted way. This means that the optimal microstructure and topography for a given chemical composition will not necessarily apply to another material with a different chemical composition.

Practical recommendations

This chapter has attempted to describe our current understanding and knowledge of surfaces, relevant to implants, and has also outlined potentials for future development. Much of this has been aimed at providing a general understanding of implant surfaces, and how they may behave and be affected in different situations. This section will address some questions of interest to the practitioner. A standard question of debate is: How "forgiving" are the oral tissues when it comes to the choice of material, surface treatment, surface purity, etc? There is no easy answer to this. We know that corroding materials (e.g. Fe) and allergenic materials (e.g. Ni and Cr) are a disaster in most cases. However, it is not known what levels of dissolved ions of these and other materials are tolerable locally or systemically. When it comes to contaminants in the monolayer – typically about 10 ng per cm^2 or less of the implant surface area – or surface atoms that do not dissolve, even less is known. One can only refer to clinical statistics and extrapolations from *in vivo* animal and *in vitro* experiments. Nevertheless, it is possible to give some general recommendations.

From a large number of non-biological applications, involving functional surfaces, it is known that impurities/contaminants on the ng/cm^2 level or less can have detrimental effects. There is every reason to believe that this could equally be true for implants, in unfortunate cases. Therefore highly standardized procedures are recommended, preferably using implants which have been hermetically sealed and sterilized at the factory. Manufacture should also involve careful process and product control using state-of-the-art surface analysis. Such implants, with well-documented, good clinical records, would serve as a reliable starting point for the clinical practitioner.

At the clinic, it is important not to contaminate the quality-controlled implant by careless handling. Today there is an unavoidable degree of uncertainty connected with manual handling of the implant and exposure to the ambient air at the clinic after opening the sterile packaging; prior to insertion into the implant site. Future functionalization; specialized coatings and/or new procedures may eventually eliminate these uncertainties.

References

[1] *Kasemo, B., Lausmaa, J.* Surface science aspects of inorganic biomaterials. CRC Crit Rev Biocomp 1986; *2:* 335–380.

[2] *Kasemo, B., Lausmaa, J.* Biomaterials and implant materials: A surface science approach. Int J Oral Maxillofac Surg 1988; *3:* 247–259.

[3] *Davies, J.E.* (Ed). The bone–biomaterial interface. Toronto: University of Toronto Press, 1991.

[4] *Smith, D. C., Pilliar, R. M., Chernecky, R.* Dental implant materials. I. Some effects of preparative procedures on surface topography. J Biomed Mater Res 1991; *25:* 1045–1068.

[5] *Smith, D. C., Pilliar, R. M., Metson, J. B., McIntyre, N. S.* Dental implant materials. II. Preparative procedures and surface spectroscopic studies. J Biomed Mater Res 1991; *25:* 1069–1084.

[6] *Lausmaa, J., Kasemo, B., Rolander, U., Bjursten, L. M., Ericson, L. E., Rosander, L., Thomsen, P.* Preparation, surface spectroscopic and electron microscopic characterization of titanium implant materials. In: *Ratner, B. D. (ed).* Surface characterization of biomaterials. pp. 161–174. New York: Elsevier; 1988.

[7] *Lausmaa, J., Kasemo, B., Mattsson, H.* Surface spectroscopic characterization of titanium implant materials. Appl Surface Sci 1990; *44:* 133–146.

[8] *Ask, M., Lausmaa, J., Kasemo, B.* Preparation and surface spectroscopic characterization of oxide films on Ti6A14V. Appl Surface Sci 1988–89; *35:* 283–301.

[9] *Lugowski, S. J., Smith, D. C., McHugh, A. D., Loon, J. C. V.* Release of metal ions from dental implant materials *in vivo:* Determination of Al, Co, Cr, Mo, Ni, V, and Ti in organ tissue. J Biomed Mater Res 1991; *25:* 1443–1458.

[10] *Sundgren, J. E., Bodö, P., Lundström, I.* Auger electron spectroscopic studies of the interface between human tissue and implants of titanium and stainless steel. J Colloid Interface Sci 1986; *110:* 9–20.

[11] *Healy, K. E., Ducheyne, P.* Oxidation kinetics of titanium thin films in model physiologic environments. J Colloid Interface Sci 1992; *150:* 404–417.

[12] *Healy, K. E., Ducheyne, P.* Hydration and preferential molecular adsorption on titanium *in vitro.* Biomaterials 1992; *13:* 553–561.

[13] *Tengvall, P., Lundström, I.* Physicochemical considerations of titanium as a biomaterial. Clin Mater 1992; *9:* 115–134.

[14] *Hanawa, T., Ota, M.* Calcium phosphate naturally formed on titanium in electrolyte solution. Biomaterials 1991; *12:* 767–774.

[15] *Thiel, P. A., Madey, T. E.* The interaction of water with solid surfaces: fundamental aspects. Surface Sci Rep 1987; *7:* 211–385.

[16] *Andrade, J. D., Hlady, V.* (ed). Protein adsorption and materials biocompatibility: a tutorial review and suggested hypotheses. Vol 79. Advances in polymer science. Washington, D.C., American Chemical Society, 1987.

[17] *Bamford, C. H., Cooper, S. L., Tsuruta, T.* (ed). The Vroman effect. Utrecht: VSP, 1992.

[18] *Brunette, D. M.* The effect of surface topography on the behaviour of cells. Int J Oral Maxillofac Implants 1988; *3:* 231–246.

Chapter 5
Part 2.

Implant systems

D. van Steenberghe

For several decades now, the rehabilitation of partial or full edentulousness by means of oral implants has been attempted; mostly unsuccessfully; by trial and error. Although there are a number of case reports, involving different implant designs, and testifying to survival times of up to 20 years or more, little scientifically documented data are available. Surveys often indicate increased losses of implants over the years, and 5 or 10 year survival rates are unacceptable for routine clinical use.

Implantable devices, such as oral implants, are not subject to premarketing evaluation. While a new drug has to be tested for years *in vitro*, in animals and in strictly supervised clinical trials before being offered to the public, many oral implants were first tried out by an individual doctor or a newly created company, on uninformed patients. Animal experiments and histological data were either non-existent or undertaken several years later, although some tentative legislation does now exist in North America. The dentist therefore needs to seek information on the different implant systems available, in order to be able to chart a path through the forest of commercialism. Patients must be provided with scientifically-based information, and not just commercial "hype".

Classification of oral implants

Oral implants are, by definition, artefacts that are put into contact with oral connective tissues. A denture is not an implant, therefore, since it is carried on an epithelialized surface. On the other hand, intramucosal retention devices inserted in superficial incisions and which are soon separated from the gingival connective tissue by an epithelial lining; can be considered as implants. The same applies to endosseous implants; which are often surrounded by a fibrous capsule and later marsupialized (i.e. epithelial downgrowth along the interface progressively separates the implant from the bone).

There are four main oral implant categories:

(1) intramucosal (no longer used);
(2) subperiosteal (rapidly declining in use);
(3) transmandibular;
(4) endosseous:
    (i)   surrounded by a fibrous capsule;
    (ii) achieving osseointegration
          (by far the most popular).

Intramucosal

This type of implant involves cutting small intramucosal retentive areas in which to place buttons attached to the denture (Fig. 1). These buttons fit directly into the retentions and, after a few days of painful healing, are completely epithelialized. Constant movement, trapped food particles and bacterial colonization result in a chronic inflammatory state, ulceration and the regular occurrence of acute abscesses.

Owing to these side-effects, the limited retention and poor short-term results, this method has been completely abandoned.

Subperiosteal implants

Here, a tailor-made metallic frame is placed on the jaw bone, and will be kept in place by the overlying periosteum. This is a two-stage procedure. An incision is made on top of the crest and the mucoperiosteum is reflected both labially and orally. Under sterile conditions, an impression is taken of the bone crest anatomy and a model cast is poured out in hard plaster. In a few days the frame, made of a biocompatible alloy, is constructed on the model; there are generally four posts to penetrate the mucoperiosteum and to support the removable denture. This frame is installed during a second surgical procedure, during which the first crestal incision is reopened, and sutured again around the four abutments. After one to several weeks of healing, the removable prosthesis is installed on top of this (Fig. 2). Subperiosteal implants can theoretically be used in both upper and lower jaws, but because of the inevitable bone resorption that results from the supra-osteal loading (because of the improved prosthetic retention; higher chewing forces are achieved)

this therapeutic approach is normally advocated for lower jaws only. Indeed, the bone resorption in the upper jaw can result in sinus or nasal cavity penetration.

Evidence has been presented for the apical migration of the gingival epithelium along the entire subperiosteal frame, which can therefore be considered as marsupialized. Infection in the pockets thus created can lead to acute discomfort or even abscess formation.

Very few documented studies are available and the success rate varies tremendously. Because of the difficulties involved in soft tissue handling when such a complication occurs, the use of subperiosteal implants has been progressively abandoned. Some authors[1] report a 93% survival rate after 5 and a 64% survival rate after 10 years, while others[2] found an average of 36% after 10 years.

Transmandibular implants

Originally described by *Small*, the so-called staple bone implant can, for obvious reasons, only be applied in the symphyseal area of the lower jaw. This technique involves general anaesthesia and an extra-oral incision under the chin. Once the lower border of the mandible has been uncovered, a series of holes are drilled in the mandibular basal bone; to receive a number of stabilizing pins. Two posts go through the entire mandibular height and through the mucoperiosteum and act as abutments to carry an overdenture (Fig. 3). The latter is only placed after a few weeks of healing. The staple is made of titanium alloy. To help the surgeon to maintain a parallel course during drilling and to avoid the mental foramina, a drill guide is available.

The transmandibular staple bone implant is

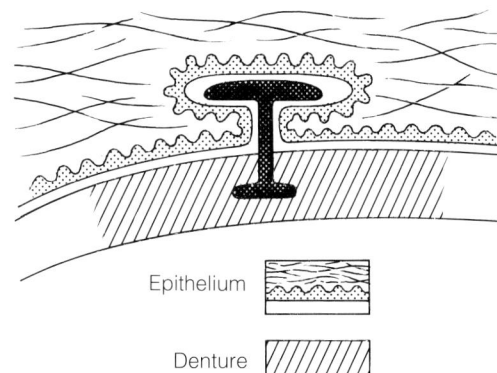

Epithelium

Denture

Fig. 1. Intramucosal "implant", completely surrounded by an epithelial lining.

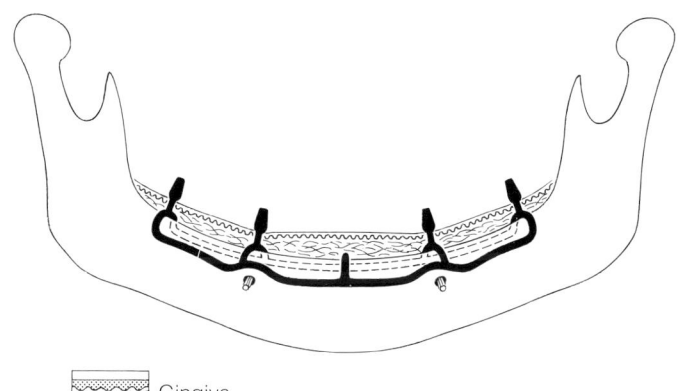

Gingiva

Fig. 2. Subperiosteal implant in the mandible. Note the localization of the saddle towards the foramina mentales and the epithelial downgrowth along the posts.

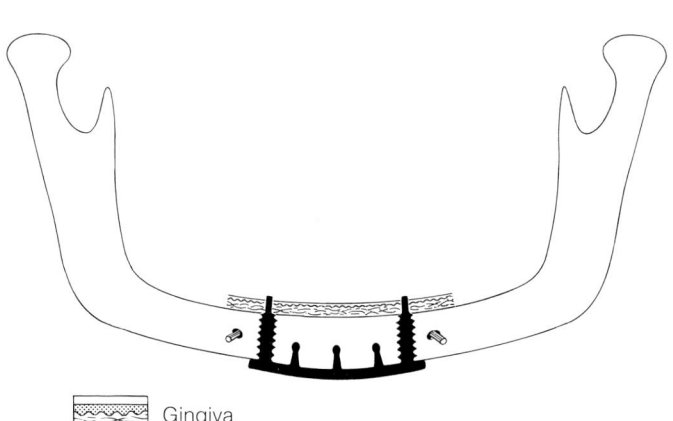

Gingiva

Fig. 3. Example of a transmandibular implant, to be placed via an extraoral incision in between the foramina mentales. Besides some stabilizing pins (here 3) two posts pierce the gingiva and can function as abutments for an overdenture.

one of the two implant systems with more than 10 years follow-up data. *Small* reported a 94% cumulative success rate after 5 years and 90% after 10 years[3]. This is one of the two oral implant systems for which documented 10-year follow-up records exist for consecutive patients and which gave good results.

A similar approach was developed in the eighties by *Bosker* in the Netherlands. Here, the implant is made of gold alloy, and is composed of a series of pieces which are screwed together. This time four posts, interconnected by a coronal bar, are available to support the overdenture. A drill guide is also available for this system, in order to achieve optimal positioning of the posts. The average success rate reported by *Bosker* after 1 to 12 years of observation was 98%[4].

In cases of implant failure, the removal of the transmandibular posts is a difficult undertaking, often resulting in significant bone loss. Another drawback of this technique is its limitation to the fully edentulous lower jaw, which means that the surgeon has to familiarize him(her)self with another implant system to deal with upper jaw defects or partial edentulism.

Endosseous systems

The variety of different implant shapes and material characteristics proposed for these systems is impressive. Many pioneers developed their own implants and tried hard to convince others of their benefits. Most did not stand the test of time. Endosseous implant systems can be divided into two categories:

(1) those that, owing to limited bone necrosis during surgery, result in encapsu-

lation of the implant by a poorly differentiated scar tissue;

(2) those that achieve osseointegration over a significant part of their surface area.

Fibrously encapsulated implants

These have a three-dimensional design and achieve a macroscopic retention; since if they had; for example; a cylindrical configuration they would easily be exfoliated by axial forces in a coronal direction.

Blade implants

Numerous different shapes have been developed. They are associated with the name of *Linkow* (New York) and are made of a wide variety of materials, ranging from Cr, Ni and Va to the more biocompatible titanium. After a crestal mucoperiosteal incision and the cutting under external or internal cooling of a trench into the jaw bone, the blade is impacted by gently hammering it into place (Fig. 4). More recently, blades have been developed which can be buried completely under the mucoperiosteum.

During a second-stage surgical procedure, after some months of healing under unloaded conditions; an abutment can be screwed on.

Most implants pierce the mucoperiosteum at once and the fixed prosthesis is supposed to be cemented on after a few weeks. The idea of this short healing period is to allow bone contact along the implant surface. No evidence is available today to show that this is a predictable phenomenon. Blade implants are best used in the

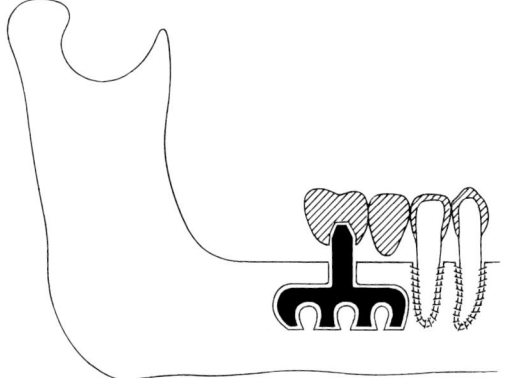

Fig. 4. A bridge is supported by a blade implant and two teeth. While the latter are anchored by organized fibre bundles of the periodontal ligament; the implant is surrounded by epithelium and scar tissue with fibres mostly parallel with the implant surface.

rehabilitation of partial edentulism where some natural teeth are present. The fibrous capsule would mimic the visco-elastic properties of the periodontal ligament.

The few reliable reports available (those with well-documented materials and methods sections, in peer-reviewed international journals) indicate a low success rate after 10 years (less than 50%)[5]. Whether recent modifications such as coatings, a two-stage procedure, improved sterility, etc., will improve these results, remains to be seen.

Disk-implant

This type of implant was developed in France by *Scortecci*. It consists of a disk with a shaft perpendicular to it. Both are introduced from the labial side after reflection of the mucoperiosteum. Two trenches are cut with a high speed bur, to receive the disk and the shaft (which pierces the gingiva at the crest); the mucoperiosteum is then closed. A fixed prosthesis can be cemented onto these shafts. This type of implant can be used in fully or partially edentulous patients and in both upper and lower jaws. Clinical results are scarce and not precisely documented so far. As in the case of blade

implants, significant bone loss results from the removal of failing implants if complications occur.

Endosseous implants showing some degree of bone contact

Most implant systems achieve this bone apposition by means of a two-stage surgical procedure; the implant is inserted into the bone and left for several months; covered by the mucoperiosteum. Some systems, however, (ITI, Ha-Ti) require a transgingival approach.

Since most commerciarely systems rely on the osseointegration principle developed by *Brånemark;* the general outline of this procedure will be described more thoroughly for the Brånemark system and only specific aspects indicated for other systems.

The Brånemark system

This implant is screw-shaped and made of c.p. titanium. It was developed as a result of basic research on bone biology per-

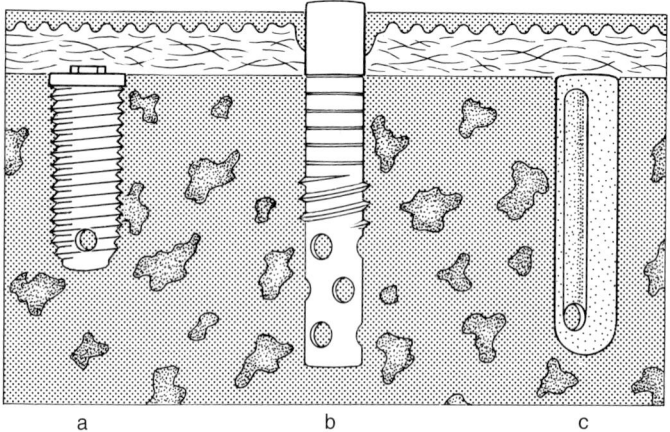

Fig. 5. Three types of two-stage endosseous implants
a: screw-shaped
b: screw/hollow-cylinder
c: cylindrical
An abutment must be attached, which will pierce the mucoperiosteum and support the prosthesis (only the middle one is in place). The drawings are only representative for available implant systems.

formed by *Brånemark* during the fifties and sixties at the universities of Lund and Gothenburg. The implant design and its surface characteristics have not been modified over more than a quarter century of clinical use, following the initial successful animal experiments.

The incision is made at some distance from the crest, in order to avoid the presence of a healing wound on top of the implants. After preparing alveoli into the bone, using relatively slow speed drills, tapping and implant insertion are done at a very slow speed (20 rpm) and copious cooling fluid is used to avoid any increase in bone temperature. Very close contact is obtained between the implant surface and the bone. A healing time of some 3–4 months is allowed for the lower jaw and 5–6 months for the upper jaw. This healing time, during which there is relative immobility at the implant/bone interface, allows the ingrowth of bone towards the grooved implant surface (Fig. 5a). At the second stage, a titanium abutment is screwed onto the top of the

implant, termed the fixture in the Brånemark system, to which the prosthesis should be attached as soon as possible. Both upper and lower, full and partial edentulism can be treated using this system. The Brånemark concept has given its name to a commercially available product, the Brånemark system. The c.p.Ti screws are available in lengths of 7–20 mm and diameters of 3–5 mm. Self-tapping screws have recently been introduced. The prosthesis is normally screwed onto the abutment.

This is by far the best documented oral implant system available, with long-term data and multi-centre studies. Characteristic of this system is that failures are mostly detected at the abutment stage or during the first 2 years of function, after which hardly any failures occur. Thus, absolute and cumulative (lifetime table calculation) success rate data are similar for the Brånemark system. Success rates of over 95% and 90% have been recorded for the lower and upper jaws, respectively.[6]

In partial edentulousness, failures are most

common in patients with a high plaque index on the remaining teeth, in locations with limited bone height (7–13 mm) or very poor bone quality, and in heavy smokers. If such factors are excluded, success rates can reach 98%[7].

In the lower jaw, two abutments connected by a Dolder bar; strictly parallel to the hinge axis to allow some tilting movement of the overdenture, offer a cheap and very reliable treatment alternative (circa 98% success, although follow-up is so far limited to less than 10 years)[8].

Removal of a failed implant does not pose a problem, just as in all other cylindrical or screw-shaped implants. The same site may even be used again, after allowing bone growth within the empty sockets created by the implants.

The IMZ system

This implant was developed in Germany by *Kirsch* in the seventies. It evolved through four different designs before the final, cylindrical; titanium, plasma sprayed and later hydroxyapatite-coated implants were launched (Fig. 5c). Unique to this two-stage implant is an inbuilt stress reducing mechanism. The system is named after this device (intra-mobile). The idea is to reduce the forces transmitted to the implant–bone interface. This reduction of impact forces does, indeed, occur, but whether it offers an advantage is still unsubstantiated. On the other hand, this device must be regularly replaced, which is time-consuming and expensive. The implants are 3.3–4 mm in diameter and 8–15 mm in length. The prosthesis is normally screwed onto the abutment. Drills for the preparation of the alveoli have an inner cooling system.

Well-documented publications on this implant type are lacking. In one publication, spanning a 10-year observation period, *Kirsch* reports that less than 5% of the implants "had to be removed". More precise data are lacking[9].

Two published reports mention an ongoing marginal bone loss (0.4 and 0.5 mm/year), which; if it does not stabilize; could lead to the loss of implants[10, 11].

The Core-Vent system

A series of different implant designs, Core-Vent, Screw-Vent, Swede-Vent and Mini-Vent have been developed by *Niznick* in the USA, during the seventies and eighties. The original Core-Vent implant consists of a hollow cylinder, threaded on the coronal part of the outer surface, and with holes in the apical region (Fig. 5b). It is made of titanium alloy and is a two-stage implant. The diameter is 4.3 and 5.3 mm and lengths vary from 8–16 mm. Drills for bone preparation have an inner cooling system.

The Screw-Vent is similar in design to the Brånemark system. Different versions include titanium alloy, c.p. titanium and hydroxyapatite coated implants. Lengths vary between 8 and 16 mm (Fig. 5a).

The Bio-Vent implant is a cylindrical, hydroxyapatite-coated implant with vertical grooves and an apical vent. As with the two previous models, this is a two-stage implant (Fig. 5c).

The clinical data are limited and only cover the short-term.

The one limited comparative study available[12] seems to indicate that although the Screw-Vent looks similar to the Brånemark system, the clinical results are different. This needs to be further substantiated before any conclusions can be drawn.

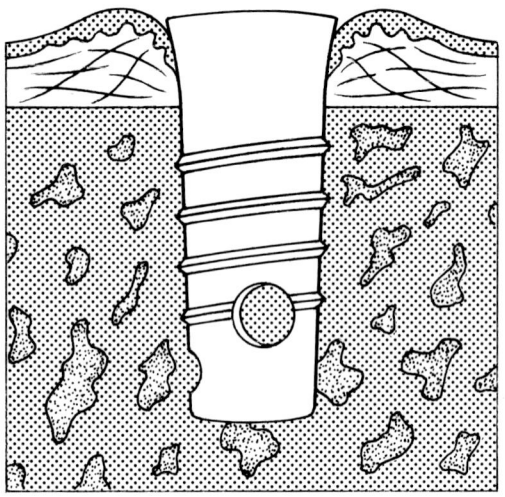

Fig. 6. One-stage hollow; cylindrical; screw-type implant.

The ITI system

In the mid-seventies *Schroeder* tried out a basket cylinder titanium plasma-sprayed implant in monkeys.

New designs have been introduced in clinical practice: hollow cylinder, hollow screw and solid screw, the surfaces of which are still plasma sprayed. The most significant feature of this implant system is that it is a one-stage procedure: the implant is not submerged (Fig. 6). The incision is thus made on the alveolar crest. The implants have holes in the apical part, and a smooth surface collar which pierces through the gingiva. The system is now known under the name Bonefit. It can be used in both jaws, in cases of both full and partial edentulism. The lengths vary between 8 and 16 mm for the one-part hollowcylinder and hollowscrew implants and between 8 and 12 mm for the two-part implants. They all have a diameter of 3.5 mm. The prostheses are screwed or cemented onto the abutments. The short-term clinical reports (3 years) indicate a high success rate (±96%)[13].

HA-Ti implants

This implant was developed by *Lederman* (who also developed the one-stage TPS screw) and has been tested clinically since 1985. It consists of a hand-driven self-tapping conical titanium screw (HA means hand and not hydroxyapatite). The diameter (at the neck) varies from 3.5–7 mm and the length from 11–20 mm. After preparation of the alveolus, the implant is inserted with a wrench, using a very low speed. It can be placed in one or in two stages. Prefabricated ceramic crowns are easily fixed on top of them. Clinical data are too scarce to draw any conclusion[14].

The Integral system

This hydroxyapatite-coated cylindrical implant was developed in the mid-eighties and has been in clinical use since then. It is a two-stage implant; inserted in the prepared alveolus by press-fit, and can receive titanium abutments (see Fig. 5c). The latter exists in different shapes to allow prosthetic superstructures screwed on or cemented on top of the abutment. Both fixed and removable prostheses can be used. The implants have a diameter of 3.25–4 mm and are available in different lengths between 4 and 15 mm.

In one 5 year observation period using cumulative success rates; the results the short-term results seem good. A total of 770 implants were placed in more than 200 patients. While after one year of loading the success rate was 99%, it fell to 95% after 4 years. Success meant that the implants did not have to be removed.[15]

The Astra system

One of the most recently developed oral implant systems is the Astra. This is a two-stage, self-tapping c.p. titanium screw, with lengths of 8–19 mm and diameters between 3.5 and 4 mm (Fig. 5a). It is similar to the Brånemark implant, but has a typical conical-shaped abutment, which by its precision fit aims to avoid leakage between implant and abutment.

The clinical importance of such leakage is unknown. The prosthesis is screwed onto the abutment. Here too, short-term clinical data (3 years) indicate excellent results (±98%)[16].

Conclusions

This far from complete review of the available oral implant systems examined the biological background and origin of the different systems, as well as their particular characteristics (material, design, surface, size). It appears that an intimate bone contact is recognized worldwide as vital for achieving long-term stability of the anchoring elements. With the exception of two systems (Brånemark and the staple bone implant of Small) no satisfactory long-term (more than 10 years) results are available for patients. However, a number of more recently introduced systems (e.g. Bonefit, Astra) have yielded excellent short-term data. The lack of organized comparative systems still leaves two questions unanswered: how significant are the different characteristics and/or how important are surgical and prosthetic skills (software)?

One should be aware of the fact that for oral implant systems, in contrast to ENT, orthopaedic or plastic surgery implants, some are used by general practitioners while others are used only by periodontists and oral surgeons. The importance of surgical skill and a team approach needs to be evaluated by comparative studies.

References

[1] *Bodine, R. L.,* and *Yanase, R. T.* 30-year report on 28 implant dentures inserted between 1952 and 1959. Int Symp on Preprosthetic Surgery. Palm Springs, CA, 16–18 May 1985.

[2] *Goldberg, N. I.* Risk of subperiosteal implants. In: *P. Schnitman* and *L. Shulman* (eds). Dental implants: benefit and risk, U.S. Dept of Health and Human Services 1980; 89–95.

[3] *Small, I. A.* Benefit and risk of mandibular staple bone plates. In: *P. Schnitman* and *L. Shulman* (eds). Dental implants: benefit and risk. U.S. Dept of Health and Human Services, NIH 1980; pp. 139–151.

[4] *Bosker, H., Van Dijk, L.* The transmandibular implant: a 12-year follow-up study. J Oral Maxillofac Surg 1989; *47:* 442–450.

[5] *Smithloff, M., Fritz, M.* The use of blade implants in a selected population of partially edentulous adults, a 15-year report. J Periodontol 1987; *58:* 589–593.

[6] *Adell, R., Eriksson, B., Lekholm, U., Brånemark, P.-I., Jemt, T.* A long-term follow-up study of osseointegrated implants in the treatment of totally edentulous jaws. Int J Oral Maxillofac Implants 1990; 347–359.

[7] *van Steenberghe, D., Lekholm, U., Bolender, C., Folmer, T., Henry, P., Herrmann, I., Higuchi, K., Laney, W., Linden, U., Astrand P.* The applicability of osseointegrated oral implants in the rehabilitation of partial edentulism: A prospective multicenter study on 558 fixtures. Int J Oral Maxillofac Implants 1990; 272–282.

[8] *Quirynen, M.* Naert, I., van Steenberghe, D., Teerlinck J., Dekeyser, C., Theuniers, G. Periodontal aspects of osseointegrated fixtures supporting an overdenture: A 4-year retrospective study. J Clin Periodontol 1991; *18:* 719–728.

[9] *Kirsch, A., Ackerman, K. L.* The IMZ osseointegrated implant system. Dent Clin North Am 1989; *33:* 733–761.

[10] *Quirynen, M., Naert, I., van Steenberghe, D., Duchateau, L., Darius, P.* Periodontal indices around osseointegrated oral implants supporting overdentures. Brussels. In: Overdentures on Oral Implants, E. Schepers. ed, Leuven University Press pp. 97–112, 1991.

[11] *Schramm-Scherer, B., Dietrich, U., Alt, K., Tetsch, P.* Untersuchungen zum Knochenabbau nach IMZ- und TPS-Implantationen im zahnlosen Unterkiefer. Z Zahnärztl Implantol 1988; *4:* 115–119.

[12] *De Bruyn, H., Collaert, B., Linden, U., Flygare, L. A..* A comparative study of the clinical efficacy of Screw-Vent implants versus Brånemark fixtures, installed in a periodontal clinic. Clin Oral Impl Res 1992; *3:* 32–41.

[13] *Buser, D., Weber, H. P., Brägger, U., Balsiger, C.* Tissue integration of one-stage ITI implants; 3-year results of a longitudinal study with hollow-screw implants. Int J Oral Maxillofac Implants 1991; *6:* 405–412.

[14] *Ledermann, Ph.* Ein universelles endossales Implantationskonzept. Swiss Dent 1988; *9:* 7–18.

[15] *Kent, J., Block, M., Finger, I., Guerra, L., Larsen, H., Misiek, D.* Biointegrated hydroxyapatite-coated dental implants: 5-year clinical observations. JADA 1990; *121:* 138–144.

[16] *Arvidson, K., Brystedt, H., Frykholm, A., von Konow, L., Lothigius, E.* A 3-year clinical study of Astra dental implants in the treatment of edentulous mandibles. Int J Oral Maxillofacial Implants 1992; *7:* 321–329.

Chapter 5
Part 3.

Software:
Surgical aspects of implant installation

F. W. Neukam, J.-E. Hausamen,
H. Schliephake

Over the past few decades, experimental research has answered a number of questions regarding tissue reactions after insertion of implants. This has led to the development of biocompatible materials and long-lasting, successful endosseous implant systems which are based on a direct structural and functional union – known as osseointegration – between the bone and the surface of the implant. The osseointegration of the foreign "implant", however, is only possible if it is made of a biocompatible material, if it provides a defined surface structure and if the shape of the implant allows a controlled load transmission to the peri-implant bone. An atraumatic surgical technique and an adequate period for bone healing and remodelling are also important elements in successful implantation.

Preconditions for the operation

Implantation may be carried out if the general health of the patient fulfils the requirements which are necessary for any kind of elective surgery. Age is not a vital factor in the selection of patients for implantation. The general physical and psychological state of the patient are rather more important.

Particular attention should be paid to the local conditions at the prospective implantation site. Among other things, retained roots, impacted teeth, cysts and; of course, infections due to diseases of the jaw bones must be treated before implantation can be performed. In brief, a successful implant operation depends on the hard and soft tissues of the jaw being intact and free from disease. Any disease could impair wound healing and bone healing and may therefore prevent the osseointegration of an implant. Significant plaque accumulation and gingival inflammation in partially edentulous patients at the time of surgery also increase the risk of implant failure. Therefore, diseases of the oral soft tissues must be treated before implantation, so that healing is completed before insertion of the implants. In the case of lesions of the mucosa a period of 4–6 weeks; and in cases of bone defects an interval of no less than 12 months; must be allowed.

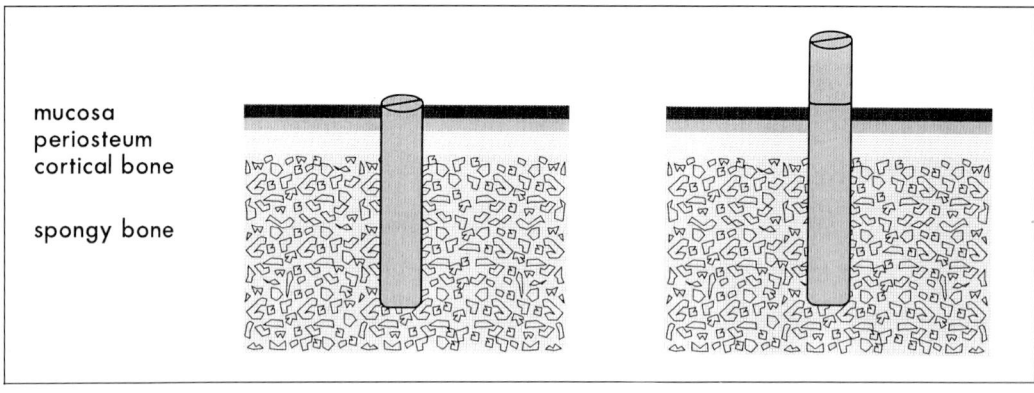

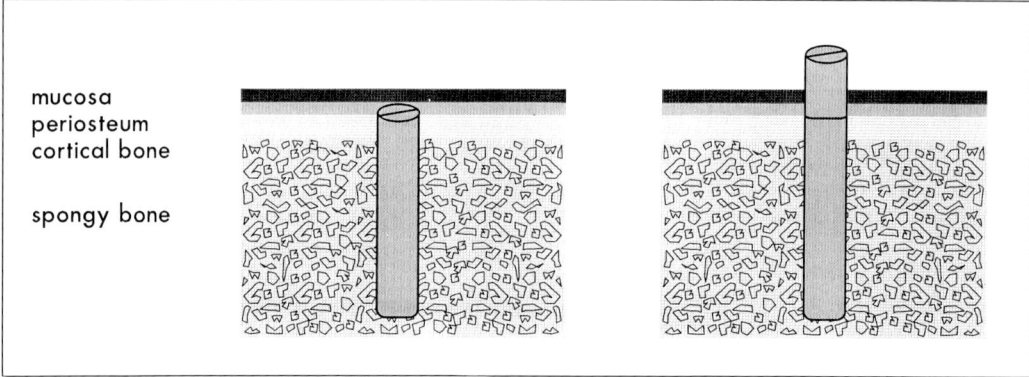

Fig. 1. Implantation procedures:

a. Submerged implants are inserted into the bone without penetrating the mucosa during the healing period of 3–6 months. In a second operation, they are re-exposed.

b. Non-submerged implants penetrate the oral mucosa during the healing period. No second operation is necessary.

Contraindications to implants

Contraindications to implantation include generalized diseases of bone, haemorrhagic diseases, diseases of the haematopoietic system, rheumatic diseases, immune deficiencies, as well as psychotic syndromes and alcohol and drug abuse. There may also be problems in certain cases of metabolic diseases involving increased risk of infections, such as in poorly controlled diabetes mellitus. After irradiation of the jaw bone, the indications for implantation must be considered carefully. Implantation should be considered, at the earliest, one year after irradiation[1]. Heavy smokers form a relative contraindication too.

Implantation procedures

Implantation techniques include both one-stage and two-stage procedures and vary with regard to the time of implantation and the onset of functional loading.

In one-stage procedures, the implants which are inserted into the bone, already penetrate the soft tissue during the healing period. Non-submerged implants need a second surgical procedure to gain access to them prior to the prosthetic treatment (Fig. 1). Conversely, in two-stage procedures, the implants are submerged under the mucosa and must be re-exposed in a second operation, following the healing phase. During the healing period of 3–6 months after insertion, submerged implants are free of functional loading forces. Functional loading commences following re-exposure of the implants and the subsequent prosthetic treatment. After implantation in a one-stage procedure, two different loading conditions are possible. In the edentulous mandible, several, usually four or more, non-submerged implants are loaded immediately after insertion. A bar-type anchoring system fixes the denture to the implants, and serves as an external splint. When fixed prostheses such as single crowns or bridges are to be used, the non-submerged implants heal without functional loading for a period of 3–6 months[2–4].

Finally, implant procedures are characterized by the time of implant insertion (Fig. 2). In this way, a distinction may be made between immediate, delayed and late implantation. The former is defined as the insertion of an implant into the empty alveolus immediately after tooth extraction. In a delayed implant placement technique, the implant is not placed immediately into the extraction socket, but 6–8 weeks later, following healing of the mucosa. In a late implantation technique, the implants are inserted into an edentulous area after bone healing of the former extraction sites. Late implantation methods are well documented, with good long-term treatment results and can be considered as routine procedures[5–7].

The advantage of an immediate or delayed implantation is thought to be the long-term preservation of the alveolar bone by functional loading, through the osseointegrated implant[8, 9]. Although preliminary results for immediate and delayed implantation techniques are promising[10, 11], long-term follow-up studies are not currently available. These procedures should, therefore, be kept for motivated exceptions. In cases of acute or subacute infection of periodontal soft tissue, delayed implantation 6–8 weeks after removal of the tooth and healing of the soft tissue is recommended; alternatively, a late implantation may be performed. In general, late implantation, the safest implant placement procedure, is preferred. In cases of acute or subacute periodontal or periapical infection or traumatic loss of alveolar bone, an implantation at least 6 months after removal of the tooth is recommended, as sufficient osseous regeneration of the extraction socket can be expected only after this period. It may be even safer to allow 12 months for bone healing, if extensive damage to the alveolar bone has occurred.

Implant-related anatomy – the mandible

During implantations in the mandible, there is a risk of damaging the inferior alveolar nerve in the mandibular canal or distal to the mental foramen in the soft tissues of the lip. The position of the mandibular canal is dependent on the degree of jaw atrophy and often describes an S-shaped curve on its way from the lingula to the mental foramen (Fig. 3). The mental foramen may be located directly on the alveolar ridge in cases of jaw atrophy. In extreme degrees of resorption, even loss of the bony roof of the mandibular

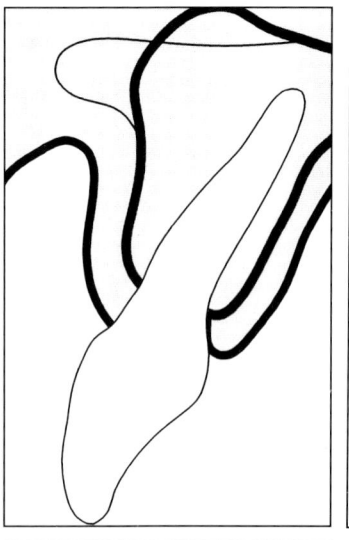
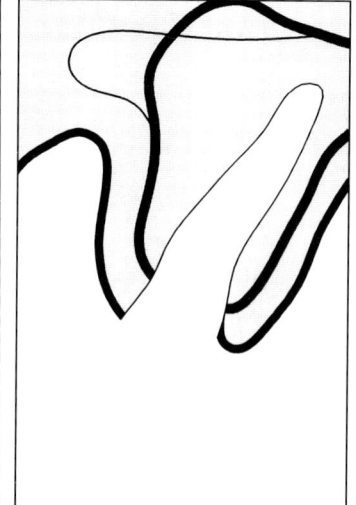
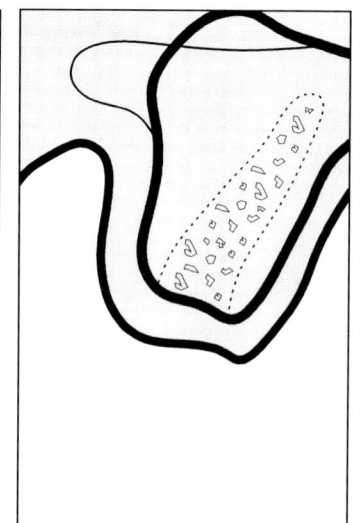

Fig. 2a

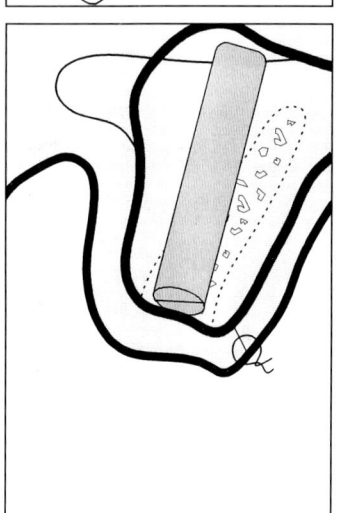

Fig. 2. Implantation procedures:
(a) In a late implantation technique, the implant is inserted into the bone 6–12 months after tooth extraction and healing of the alveolus.
(b) In a delayed implantation procedure, the implant is placed into the bone 6–8 weeks after tooth extraction and healing of the mucosa.
(c) In an immediate placement technique, the implant is placed into the bone immediately after tooth extraction.

canal has been described, so that the neurovascular bundle is situated directly on the alveolar ridge.[12]

Apart from the residual bone height, the location of the inferior alveolar nerve is the limiting factor for implantations in the posterior part of the edentulous atrophic jaw. The exposure and relocation of the neurovascular bundle may prevent an implantation into the mandible in extreme cases of atrophy[13, 14].

Reliable prosthesis stabilization can be achieved by insertion of 2–6 implants in the interforaminal region of the jaw bone in combination with an overdenture or a removable hybrid prosthesis or – with a fixed

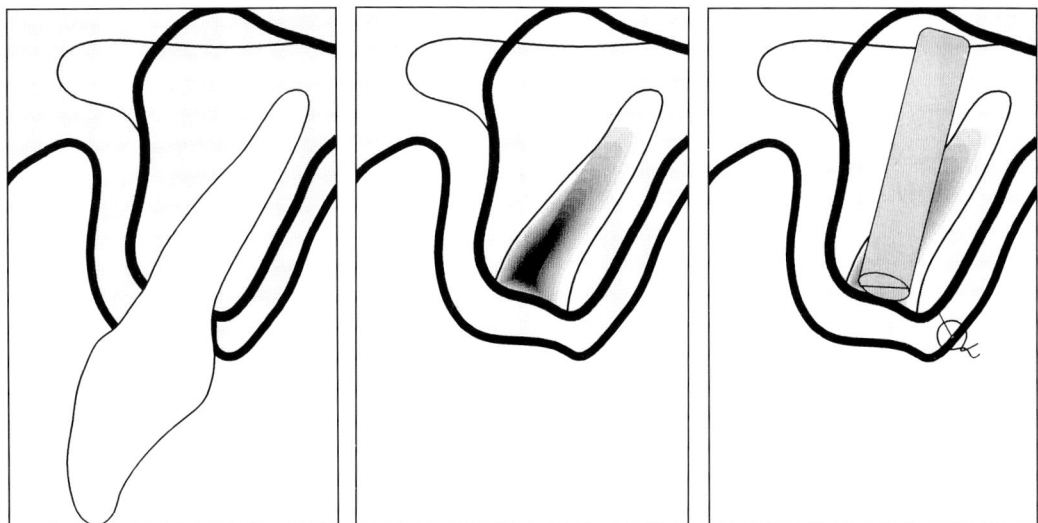

Fig. 2b

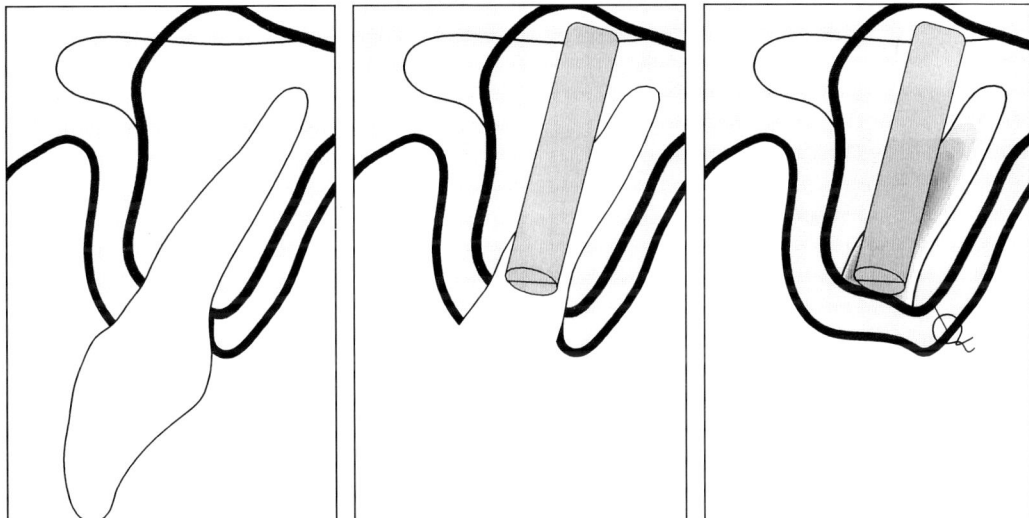

Fig. 2c

prosthesis in cases of moderate atrophy, and a vertical bone height of 10–15 mm, provided the mental foramen is not situated on the alveolar ridge and that pressure on the mental nerve can be avoided.

In cases of marked atrophy, and with the neurovascular bundle situated on the alveolar ridge and a vertical residual height of 6–10 mm, restoration with a resilient overdenture is contraindicated. By loading not only the implants, but also the denture-bearing soft tissue, irritation of the mental nerve by the prosthesis occurs.

Patients with a mandibular vertical height of only 5–6 mm at the symphysis may be

91

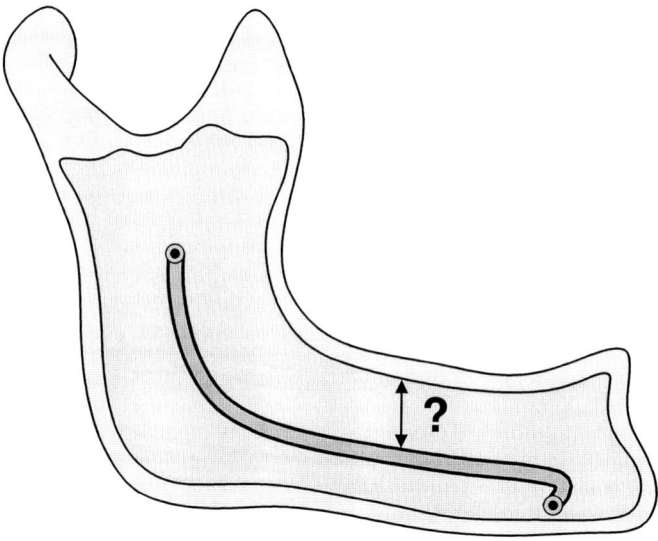

Fig. 3. In the mandibular posterior region, implant placement is difficult owing to the presence of the inferior alveolar nerve. Radiographic measurement is necessary to determine the bone height from the crestal bone to the canal.

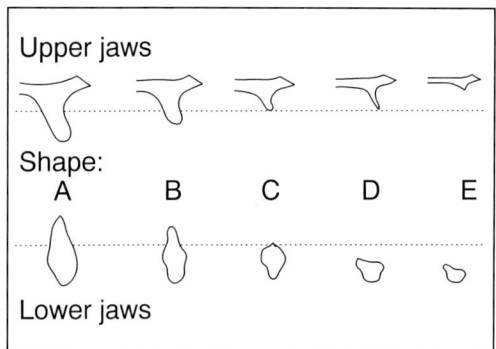

Fig. 4a

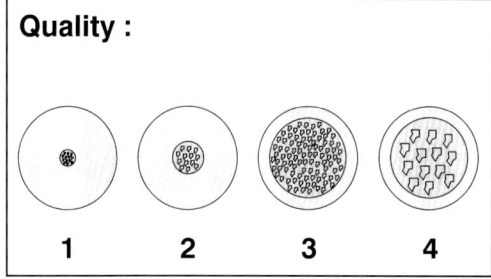

Fig. 4b

Fig. 4. Morphology and quality of the jaw bone[38].
(a) Resorption patterns in the anterior region of the maxilla and mandible. A: minimal or no bone resorption, B: moderate bone resorption, C: severe bone resorption with only basal bone remaining, D+E: progressively severe resorption into basal bone.
(b) Cortical and cancellous bone quality classifications:
1: majority of residual bone consists of cortical bone; 2: a thick cortical layer surrounds spongy bone; 3: a thin layer of cortical bone surrounds spongy bone; 4: a thin layer of cortical bone surrounds low density spongy bone.

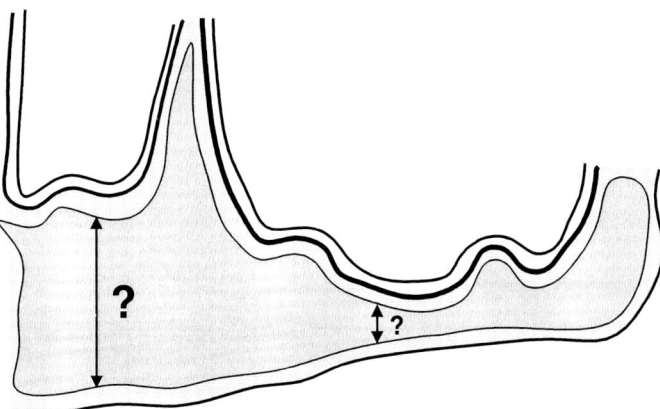

Fig. 5. In the maxilla, implantation can be difficult owing to the presence of the nasal cavity and sinus floor. Measurements are necessary in order to determine the bone height from the crestal bone to the nasal cavity or sinus floor.

candidates for bone grafting techniques in combination with implants (Fig. 4).

Implant-related anatomy – the maxilla

Implantations in the fully edentulous maxilla are less often required. However, they may be necessary in cases of extreme jaw atrophy or a pronounced gag reflex. Perforation into the nasal cavity or the maxillary sinus during the preparation of the implant site is not a rarity, as the location of the nasal floor and the maxillary sinus cannot clearly be seen in radiography unless CT scans are taken (Fig. 5). In the case of a perforation into the maxillary sinus, an implantation is still considered to be justified if primary stability of the implant is achieved after the preparation of the implant site, if the mucosal lining of the maxillary sinus or of the nasal floor has not been violated and if the implant extends no more than 0.5–1 mm beyond the osseous floor. The complete closure of the perforation by the implants may be one reason, since complete osseous regeneration of the defects occurs during the healing period of osseointegrated implants. Penetration of oral bacteria into the maxillary sinus can therefore be safely avoided [15, 16].

Taking into account the higher failure rate of the short implants (7 mm) used in the maxilla compared to the longer implants (10–13 mm) [17], there is more often an indication for reconstruction procedures using bone grafts and implants in the severely resorbed maxilla than in the mandible (vertical bone height of only 5–6 mm).

Sterile operating conditions

Implantations must be performed under sterile conditions. To ensure this, surgical conditions and experienced staff must be provided in the hospital or consulting room. In particular, this implies sterile surgical dress, gloves, drapes and instruments. After scrubbing, the surgeon and the surgical nurse put on sterile gowns and sterile surgical gloves. The surgical nurse arranges a sterile working field with the aid of an assisting nurse. The instruments, the implants and the covering materials are arranged on a sterile instrument tray.

The patient is prepared by disinfecting the skin of the face, chin and neck, as well as the mucosal lining of the oral cavity, using a sterile gauze pad soaked with disinfectant. The patient is then covered with sterile drapes.

Peri-operative antibiotics

During the planning of implant surgery, one must remember that all operations are performed in the bacteria-laden environment of the oral cavity, so that wounds become contaminated by bacteria of the commensal oral flora. This increases the danger of a subsequent wound infection. There is, of course, also the danger of a local infection of the peri-implant hard and soft tissues, leading to possible infection-related implant loss.

Risk factors during surgery

According to *Topazian*[18], the risks that may occur during the insertion of implants can be classified into:

(1) Host factors;
(2) Implant factors;
(3) Microbial factors;
(4) Surgical factors.

Host factors

During an incision, and particularly during the insertion of implants, the integrity of the body surface and the vascular supply is disturbed or interrupted. Systemic factors which may increase the risks of infection include advanced age[19], metabolic diseases (particularly diabetes mellitus),

obesity, steroid therapy, malnutrition and the presence of an infection elsewhere in the body.

Implant factors

Basically, any foreign material may help cause a local infection, since the local tissue defence is impaired for a prolonged period by the presence of the implant. The reactions of the soft and hard tissues following implantation have already been reported elsewhere.

Microbial factors

The probability of a bacterial infection occurring is determined by the number and the virulence of the bacteria on the one hand and by the condition of the host's defense systems on the other. The risk of infection is increased in the presence of one or more of the abovementioned systemic factors. Basically, bacteria may penetrate the surgical wound through the incision, even after local disinfection. According to *Topazian*[19], the risk of infection can be estimated to be approximately 2% in clean-contaminated surgical wounds inside the oral cavity. Although the risk of infection is, therefore, not very high, it must be taken into account that the loss of an implant implies additional costs and may require a reimplantation. Furthermore, one has to consider, that in patients with partial edentulism a high degree of plaque accumulation and associated gingival inflammation during implant surgery has caused a high implant failure rate[20]. These findings can be explained as a result of bacterial contamination during surgery[17]. In orthopaedic surgery it is well known that under aseptic operating conditions, for instance in hip surgery, bacteria of low virulence may enter the wound. This can cause late implant failure due to early low-grade infection[21]. In general, the surgical wound which is created during an implantation can be compared to a clean-contaminated wound of the respiratory or gastrointestinal tract. Therefore, even under the favourable local conditions in the oral cavity, depending on the vascularization of the jaw bones and the soft tissues, antibiotic prophylaxis during implant therapy may be indicated.

For this reason, *Topazian*[18] recommends the prophylactic administration of antibiotics in intra-oral implantations. It is always necessary in the presence of any of the systemic factors mentioned earlier.

A peri-operative prophylactic administration of antibiotics is also always necessary in osseoplastic reconstructions in combination with implants, in order not to jeopardize the bone graft[18, 22]. When bone grafting is performed, it must also be borne in mind that surgery is more extensive and longer-lasting, thereby increasing the risk of infection.

avoided, because it can have significant effects on biocompatibility[23]; (See Chapter 5.1).

Surgical implant procedures are very technique-sensitive, especially when small implants are used in a limited amount of bone. Therefore, osseointegration can be achieved only if the implant site is properly prepared, with the aid of a standardized set of instruments, creating an optimal fit with maximal contact between the bone and the entire surface of the implant. As stated earlier, the initial stability of the implant following insertion is of the utmost importance.

The temperature within the bone during cutting and drilling procedures at the implant site must not exceed 47 °C for 1 minute, otherwise thermal damage and bone tissue necrosis will occur[24, 25]. This leads to an increased risk of infection, delayed wound healing, regenerative bone resorption and possible failure of osseointegration. To avoid thermal damage, limited drilling speed under low pressure, a graduated series of sharp drills, and copious external irrigation with sterile saline solution are necessary. A flow of at least 50 ml/minute should be used. Internal irrigation is equally effective[26].

Atraumatic surgical technique

The preparation of the intra-oral soft tissues and the jaw bones must be performed precisely and as atraumatically as possible, so that the bone wound will be repaired by highly differentiated bone tissue and not by poorly differentiated scar tissue at the interface. It is not the alloplastic material alone which is important for the contact of bone to the implant surface after healing. During surgery, the clean sterile implant surface must not be allowed to come into contact with other materials. Contamination must be

Pre-operative examination

A decision can only be made as to whether implantation is possible and indicated (see Chapter 4), following clinical evaluation of the soft tissues, the periodontal status of the remaining teeth and radiographic examination of bone morphology combined with an analysis of plaster casts.

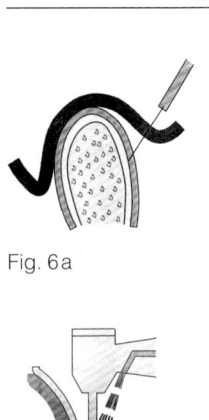
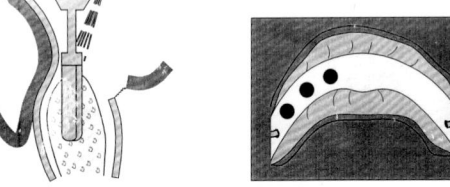

Fig. 6a

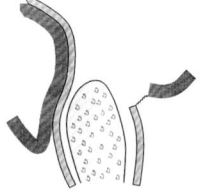
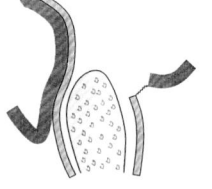
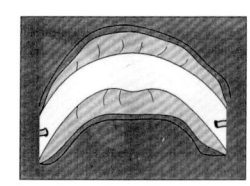

Fig. 6b

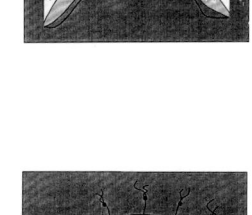

Fig. 6c

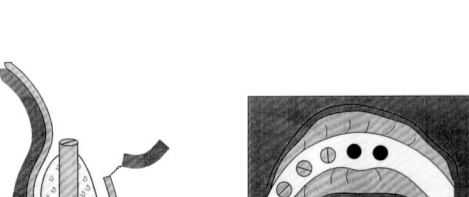
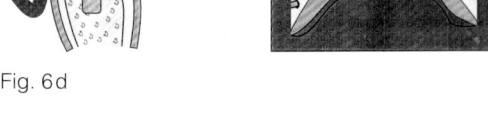

Fig. 6d

Fig. 6. Surgical technique in the edentulous mandible: implant installation.

(a) Incision through the mucosal tissues.

(b) The mucoperiosteal flap is reflected lingually and the alveolar bone is exposed.

(c) During preparation of the implant sites; copious saline irrigation is required to avoid thermal damage to the bone.

(d–e) After implant placement, the mucoperiosteal flap is sutured to achieve primary closure.

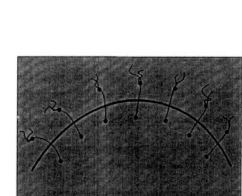

Fig. 6e

Surgical techniques

Late implantation

The most frequent indication for the insertion of endosseous implants is the edentulous atrophic mandible where 2, 4 or 5–6 implants are inserted, preferably in the interforaminal region, depending on whether an implant-supported removable denture or an implant-supported fixed bridge is planned. In addition to the edentulous maxilla and the partially edentulous jaw, a further indication is extreme atrophy of the jaw bones.

The surgical implantation technique is explained below, using the mandible and a two-stage procedure, as one example (Fig. 6).

Before the operation, the patient is asked to rinse the mouth several times with 0.1% chlorhexidine solution. The operation site is disinfected and the patient is covered with sterile drapes. Local anaesthesia includes anaesthetic block of the inferior alveolar nerve on both sides at the mandibular foramen and the buccal nerve on both sides.

Soft tissue incision

A lip retractor is used to display the site of operation. A curvilinear incision is made in the mucosa, 8–10 mm, from and parallel to the remaining alveolar ridge of the mandible, from approximately the first bicuspid region, in the vestibule of the mouth. To avoid damage to the mental nerve, this should be exposed and clearly identified. The periosteum is then incised a few millimetres from the alveolar crest and a lingually pedicled mucoperiosteal flap is dissected. The dissection is continued subperiosteally to the mental foramen, so that the mental nerve is preserved safely from both sides. Thin, sharp edges of bone must be removed with forceps.

Bone preparation

If a surgical template is to be used to identify the implantation sites, this is inserted and the implant sites are marked using a small round bur with a maximum speed of 2000 revolutions/minute. During the definition of the implantation sites, the bur penetrates the cortical bone, through to the cancellous bone underneath. In this way, the surgeon gains valuable information about the thickness of the compact bone and the quality of the cancellous bone from the mechanical resistance of the bone tissue. Usually, 2, 4 or 5–6 implants are inserted between the two mental foramina.

To keep thermal damage to a minimum during the definition of the implantation sites, and also during the later steps of the procedure, drilling is performed at low pressure, under continuous irrigation with sterile physiological sodium chloride solution. Moving the bur up and down allows the cooling agent to reach the cutting edges of the bur.

The direction of drilling of the implantation sites should be optimal with regard to the alveolar ridge of the opposite jaw and perfectly vertical in a mesio-distal direction. To achieve this, it may be desirable to start with the preparation of the distal implantation site on the left-hand side. Control is best gained by means of a direction indicator, which is inserted into the first drill-hole. The same procedure is performed with the subsequent implantation sites to the right. Attention should be paid to keeping the direction of drilling parallel in all planes to the direction indicator, which has already been placed. To achieve this, close control and good cooperation within the team are necessary. During the subsequent preparation of the remaining implantation sites from left to right, using different burs from the standardized set of instruments, the depth of the implantation site is defined by means of standardized drills according to the local bone height; care should be taken not to perforate the jaw bone on the lingual side.

If the jaw bone provides a thick cortical lamella and the cancellous bone structure is strong, it is not always necessary to extend the preparation into the opposite cortical lamella, as the jaw bone is firm enough to provide initial stability for the implants and enough resistance against functional loading forces later. In cases of a thin cortical lamella and a loose, weak cancellous bone structure, it is necessary to deepen the preparation until the opposite cortical lamella is engaged, in order to increase the stability of the implant. Endosseous implants are best placed slightly below or near the crest, to protect them from forces transmitted by the overlying removable prosthesis.

Insertion

There are three types of insertion: blade

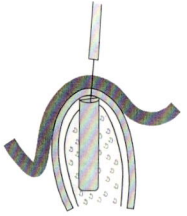

Fig. 7a

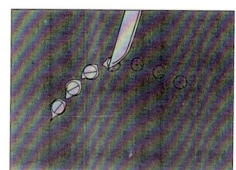

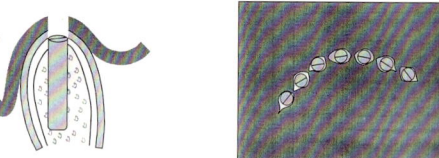

Fig. 7b

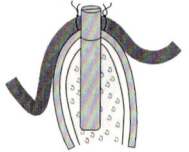

Fig. 7c

Fig. 7. Surgical technique in the edentulous mandible: abutment connection.
(a) After locating the implant, an incision is made across the implant.
(b) The mucoperiosteal layer is removed to uncover the implant.
(c) An abutment is fixed to the implant.

implants are gently hammered in until they bind, root forms are tapped into implantation sites with a press-fit, and threaded root forms are screwed into position.

Soft tissue closure

Following implant placement, the site of operation has to be cleared of bone chips and rinsed with sterile saline solution. The closure of the soft tissue must be carried out with great care, without interfering with vascularization. Relaxing periosteal incisions may contribute to tension-free mucosal closure. The patient is discharged after routine instructions and the sutures are removed after 7–10 days.

After 10–14 days at the earliest, the patient may wear his/her denture again. Prior to this, it must be carefully modified by relieving the fitting surface and adding a soft lining material. The patient is instructed not to use the denture and to see the dentist if there is any sign of pressure ulcers. A continuous check for pressure ulcers is necessary in order to avoid irritation of the

covering soft tissues. Furthermore, loading of the implants by a denture must be prevented during the healing period.

Abutment connection

In a two-step implantation procedure, the abutment connection is performed in a second operation under local anaesthesia; after a healing period of 3 months in the mandible or 6 month after implant installation in the maxilla (Fig. 7). Before this, the patient is asked to rinse the mouth several times with 0.1% chlorhexidine solution. The operation site is disinfected and the patient is covered with sterile drapes.

To uncover the implants, their exact location must be determined. A photograph, taken during the insertion of the implants, may be useful for this purpose. However, the surgeon can locate the implants by palpation of the mandibular alveolar ridge and mark the positions with a dental probe or a knife. The mucosa is opened over the implants by incisions and each implant is uncovered; the abutments are then attached. After healing of the peri-implant soft tissues, 2–4 weeks later, the prosthetic treatment may be started (see Chapter 5.4 "Prosthetic aspects").

Delayed implantation

Delayed implantation 6–8 weeks after tooth extraction is recommended if the periodontal tissues at the site of implantation are infected or damaged by trauma. In this case, the alveolar ridge is exposed by dissecting and mobilizing a buccally pedicled mucoperiostal flap. The rest of the procedure is exactly as described below for immediate implantation.

Immediate implantation

The extraction of a decayed tooth must be performed carefully in order to avoid damage to the bone at the prospective site of implantation. First, the marginal periodontal fibres are separated by a fibrotome or desmotome. Then, the soft tissues of the marginal periodontium are excised in a circular manner, so that the pocket epithelium is completely removed. Damage or fracture of the buccal wall of the alveolus must be avoided at all costs during the extraction of the tooth.

The empty extraction socket is then carefully curetted so that no granulation tissue or periodontal ligament remains in the socket. To determine the site and direction of implantation, a pre-operatively prepared template is inserted. The following steps correspond to the surgical technique used in the edentulous jaw (see above). After the implant has been inserted in a two-stage procedure, a broad-based, buccally pedicled mucoperiostal flap is dissected, thus achieving tension-free wound closure

and safe soft tissue coverage of the implantation site. In a one-stage implantation technique, the soft tissue is adapted to the implant by sutures.

In those cases where an implant is directly inserted into a fresh extraction socket, the configuration of the alveolar process must be taken into consideration. It must be ascertained that the implant can be inserted into the bone beyond the bottom of the extraction socket in order to achieve reliable initial stability of the implant. In order to avoid impairment of the aesthetics of the future restoration, it is often recommended that the implant be placed in a vertical position rather than a proclined position. Often, there is no congruity between the former extraction socket and the implant in the coronal parts of the implant, thus leaving a gap if the diameter of the implant is smaller. In such cases, it is appropriate to use autogenous bone chips, harvested from the jaw bone at a different location inside the oral cavity (area of the mentum or retromolar area of the maxilla or mandible) and inserted between the implant and the wall of the extraction socket. Furthermore, a membrane technique (see later, Guided Tissue Regeneration (GTR)) may be used to achieve guided tissue regeneration around the implant.

Treatment of the patient with extreme jaw atrophy

There are several statements in the literature about the residual height and residual width of the jaw bone necessary for implantation (Fig. 8). Insertion of implants can be performed with a high degree of safety up to a vertical residual bone height of 6–7 mm and a width of 4 mm[27–29]. In cases of bone atrophy, bone volume may be insuf-

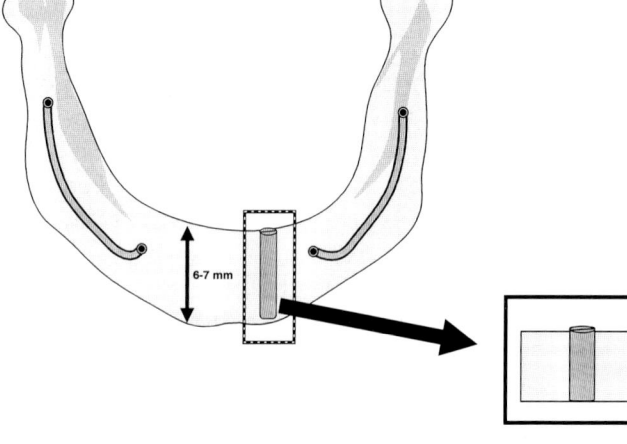

Fig. 8. In cases of severe bone resorption, installation of implants can be performed up to a vertical bone height of 6–7 mm. Implantation is considered to be justified even after perforation of the inferior cortex in the mandible.

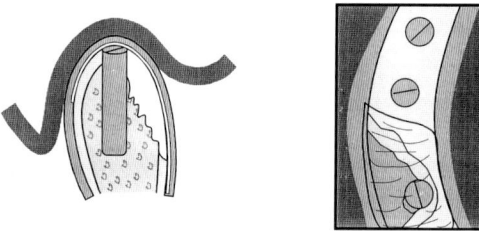

Fig. 9. Dehisced implant site covered with a membrane for guided bone tissue regeneration.

ficient to assure primary stability and osseointegration of the implant. In such cases, ridge augmentation procedures become necessary. Augmentation of bone volume can be achieved by GTR or by bone grafting techniques.

Augmentation of bone volume

Guided tissue regeneration

The principle of guided tissue regeneration is based on the assumption that different types of cells which play a role in the regeneration of bone defects have differing proliferation kinetics. During healing of os-

seous jaw defects, mesenchymal cells originating from the subepithelial connective tissue compete with cells from the osseous tissue in the differentiation of granulation tissue[30-33]. Fibroblasts and other connective tissue cells from the vicinity of the defect should be prevented from growing into the defect by covering it with a semi-permeable membrane such as an e-PTFE membrane (e.g. Gore-Tex®, WL Gore, Flagstaff, Arizona, USA). The membrane has a double function: to create a space and to act as a barrier. This should enable those cells with osseogenetic determination and which exhibit a lower proliferation rate to colonize the defect first (Fig. 9). Although preliminary human clinical applications of guided tissue regeneration technique have shown encouraging results in treating dehisced implant sites and in regeneration and enlargement techniques of jaw bone prior to implantation[34], the procedure is restricted to small bone defects. Several basic questions are still to be answered and long-term results are required prior to universal application of the technique during implantations and for bone regeneration in larger defects. On the one hand, suitable materials are not available to keep open the space which is provided by the membrane. Currently, no stable membranes are available to surround a defined space and, so far, the maximum size of the defect which can be filled by guided tissue regeneration is unknown.

Bone grafting in combination with implants

Even today, autogenous bone is still considered the material of choice for augmentation of bone volume. However, because of the potential morbidity of the donor site, there is a need for other augmentation graft materials, i.e. allogenic and xenogenic bone, bone substitutes, or proteins capable of inducing new bone formation. Further investigations are necessary to solve the problems of immunogenicity, biocompatibility, stability, and bone induction before these materials will be accepted in routine clinical practice.

Autogenous bone is available as free or microvascular pedicled grafts for augmentation of the atrophic jaw or for the reconstruction of the jaw bone in combination with implants.

Uneventful healing of a free autogenous bone graft depends on good vascularization of the recipient site, firm fixation of the graft to the underlying host bone and intimate contact between the graft surface and the overlying soft tissue.

If these conditions are fulfilled, proliferation of osteoblasts and early formation of woven bone as well as the transition to the later stage of bone induction will occur. If the recipient site is well vascularized, free bone grafts from the iliac crest are generally used for reconstruction of the jaw bone.

If extreme jaw atrophy has been found radiographically, such that the vertical residual bone height is 6–7 mm or that resorption has reached the mental spine in the mandible or the nasal spine in the maxilla, further examinations of the bone structure and morphology at the site of implantation (e.g. computed tomograms or CT-scans) are essential before the decision for an implantation in combination with a bone graft can be made.

The atrophic maxilla or mandible may be augmented by a free bone graft from the iliac crest, fixed to the local residual bone with the aid of implants (Fig. 10). Clinical results suggest that bone grafting in combination with implant installation limits resorption rates when adequately loaded[29, 35].

Bone graft augmentation of the maxillary sinus floor

After loss of teeth in the maxilla, the alveolar process undergoes resorption and the floor of the maxillary sinus moves downwards so that the thin compact bone of the sinus floor fuses with that of the alveolar process[36]. Problems may result if the thickness of the sinus floor is inadequate for stable anchorage of implants (Fig. 11). In such cases, bone grafting for sinus floor augmentation allows the creation of appropriate conditions for the insertion of implants[37].

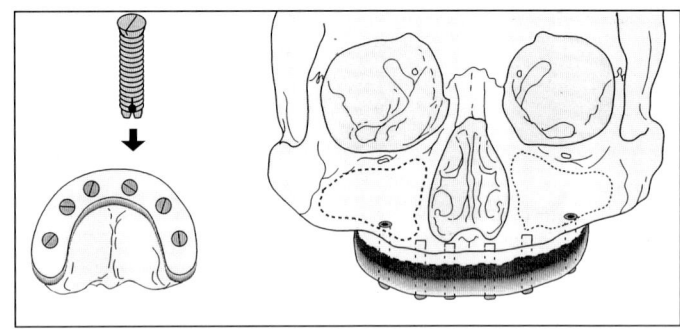

Fig. 10. In the severe resorbed maxilla or mandible, autogenous bone grafting in combination with implants is indicated. The free bone graft is fixed to the residual bone by the implants.

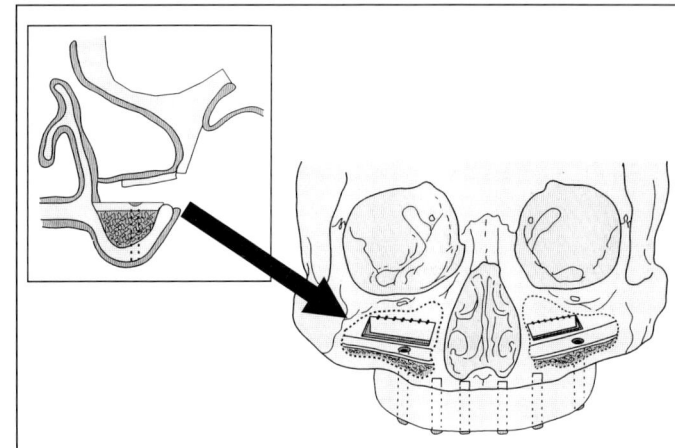

Fig. 11. In the severely resorbed posterior maxilla it may be necessary to augment the sinus floor by an autogenous bone graft before implant insertion is possible.

Summary

Over the past few decades, basic research and clinical long-term studies have proved the feasibility of the principle of osseointegration for the anchorage of implants in the jaw bones. The possibilities and limitations of this technique with regard to permanent mechanical implant stability, however, depend on the fact that the bone itself is a highly differentiated tissue. That is why implants can only become osseointegrated if the insertion is performed with great care, using an atraumatic surgical technique. The surgical aspects of implant installation therefore have a profound influence on the success or failure of osseointegration.

References

[1] *Jacobsson, M., Tjellström, A., Thomsen, P., Albrektsson, T., Turesson, I.* Integration of titanium implants in irradiated bone. Histological and clinical study. Ann Otol Rhinol Laryngol 1988; *97:* 337–340.

[2] *Sutter, F., Schroeder, A., Buser, D. A.* The new concept of ITI hollow-cylinder and hollow-screw implants: Part 1. Engineering and design. Int J Oral Maxillofac Implants 1988; *3:* 161–172.

[3] Buser, D. A., Schroeder, A., Sutter, F., Lang, N. P. The new concept of ITI hollow-cylinder and hollow-screw implants: Part 2. Clinical aspects, indications, and early clinical results. Int J Oral Maxillofac Implants 1988; 3: 173–181.

[4] Buser, D., Weber, H. P., Brägger, U., Balsiger, C. Tissue integration of one-stage ITI implants: 3-year results of a longitudinal study with hollow-cylinder and hollow-screw implants. Int J Oral Maxillofac Implants 1991; 6: 405–412.

[5] Adell, R., Lekholm, U., Rockler, B., Brånemark, P.-I. A 15-year study of osseointegrated implants in treatment of edentulous jaw. Int J Oral Surg 1981; 6: 387–416.

[6] Albrektsson, T. Knochengewebsreaktionen. In: Brånemark, P.-I., Zarb, G. A., Albrektsson T. (Hrsg.): Gewebeintegrierter Zahnersatz. pp. 129–143. Berlin: Quintessenz, 1985.

[7] Albrektsson, T., Zarb, G. A., Worthington, D. P., Eriksson, R. A. The long-term efficacy of currently used dental implants. A review and proposed criteria of success. Int J Oral Maxillofac Implants 1986; 1: 11–25.

[8] Schulte, W. Klinische und wissenschaftliche Aspekte des Einzelzahnimplantates. Erweiteres Autoreferat. Z Zahnärztl Implantol 1987; 3: 135–136.

[9] Lazzara, R. Immediate implant placement into extraction sites: Surgical and restorative advantages. Int J Periodontal Restor Dent 1989; 9: 333–343

[10] Krump, J. L., Barnett, B. G. The immediate implant: A treatment alternative. Int J Oral Maxillofac Implants 1991; 6: 19–23

[11] Tollman, D. E., Keller, E. E. Endosseous implant placement immediately following dental extraction and alveoloplasty: Preliminary report with 6-year follow-up. Int J Oral Maxillofac Implants 1991; 6: 24–28.

[12] Gabriel, A. C. Some anatomical features of the mandible. J Anat 1958; 92: 580–586.

[13] Davis, W. H., Rydevik, B., Lundborg, G., Danielsen, N., Hausamen, J.-E., Neukam, F. W. Mobilisation of the inferior alveolar nerve to allow placement of osseointegrated implants. In: Worthington, P., Brånemark, P.-I. (eds). Advanced osseointegration surgery: Applications in the maxillofacial region. pp. 129–144. Chicago: Quintessence, 1992.

[14] Rosenquist, B. Implant placement posterior to the mental foramen with transpositioning of the inferior alveolar nerve. Int J Oral Maxillofac Implants 1992; 7: 45–50.

[15] Brånemark, P.-I., Adell, R., Albrektsson, T., Lekholm, U., Lindström, J., Rockler, B. An experimental and clinical study of osseointegrated implants penetrating the nasal cavity and maxillary sinus. J Oral Maxillofac Surg 1984; 42: 497–505.

[16] Hessling, K. H., Neukam, F. W., Scheller, H., Günay, H., Schmelzeisen, R. Die extreme Atrophie des Ober- und Unterkiefers. Klinische Gesichtspunkte bei der Versorgung mit enossalen Implantaten. Z Zahnärztl Implantol 1990; 4: 35–39.

[17] van Steenberghe, D., Lekholm, U., Bolender, C., Folmer, T., Henry, P., Herrmann, I., Higuchi, K., Laney, W., Linden, U., Astrand, P. The applicability of osseointegrated oral implants in the rehabilitation of partial edentulism: A prospective multicenter study on 558 implants. Int J Oral Maxillofac Implants 1990; 5: 272–281.

[18] Topazian, R. G. The basis of antibiotic prophylaxis. In: Worthington, P., Brånemark, P.-I. (eds). Advanced osseointegration surgery: Applications in the maxillofacial region. pp. 57–66. Chicago: Quintessence, 1992.

[19] Gardner, I. D. The effect of aging on susceptibility to infection. Rev Infect Dis 1980; 2: 801–810.

[20] Haannaes, H. R. Implants and infection with special reference to oral bacteria. J Clin Periodontol 1990; 17: 516–524.

[21] Hirschmann, J. V. Antibiotics in the prevention of infection associated with prosthetic devices. In: Sugarman, B., Young, E. J. (eds). Infections associated with prosthetic devices. p 269. Boca Raton, Fla: CRC Press, 1983.

[22] Newman, M. G., Flemming, T. F. Bacteria – host interactions. In: Worthington, P., Brånemark, P.-I. (eds). Advanced osseointegration surgery: Applications in the maxillofacial region. pp. 67–79. Chicago: Quintessence, 1992.

[23] Baier, R. E., Meyer, A. E. Future directions in surface preparation of dental implants. J Dent Educ 1988; 52: 788–791.

[24] Lentrodt, J., Bull, H. G. Tierexperimentelle Untersuchungen zur Frage der Knochenregeneration nach Bohrvorgängen im Knochen. Dtsch Zahnärztl Z 1976; 31: 115–124.

[25] Eriksson, A. R. Heat-induced bone tissue injury. (Thesis) Göteborg, 1984.

[26] Kirschner, V. H., Meyer, W. Entwicklung einer Innenkühlung für chirurgische Bohrer. Dtsch Zahnärztl Z 1975; 30: 436–438.

[27] Brånemark, P.-I. Osseointegration and its experimental background. J Prosthet Dent 1983; 49: 399–410.

[28] Neukam, F. W., Scheller, H., Günay, H. Experimentelle und klinische Untersuchungen zur Auflagerungsosteoplastik in Kombination mit enossalen Implantaten. Z Zahnärztl Implantol 1989; 5: 235–241.

[29] Neukam, F. W., Hausamen, J.-E., Scheller, H. Functional and esthetic rehabilitation with Brånemark implants following oncologic surgery. In: Albrektsson, T., Zarb, G. A. (eds). The Brånemark osseointegrated implant. pp. 147–162. Chicago: Quintessence, 1989.

[30] Andreasen, J. O., Rud, J. Modes of healing histologically after endodontic surgery in 70 cases. Int J Oral Surg 1972; 1: 148–160.

[31] Dahlin, C., Gottlow, J., Linde, A., Nyman, S. Healing of maxillary and mandibular bone defects using a membrane technique. An experimental study in monkeys. Scand J Plast Reconstr Hand Surg 1990; 24: 13–19.

[32] *Seibert, J., Nyman, S.* Localized ridge augmentation in dogs: A pilot study using membranes and hydroxyapatite. J Periodontol 1990; *61:* 157–165.

[33] *Becker, J., Neukam, F. W., Schliephake, H.* Restoration of the maxillary sinus bone plate using the principle of guided tissue regeneration and a collagen type I membrane. Int J Oral Surg 1992; *21:* 243–246.

[34] *Jovanovic, S. A., Spiekermann, H., Richter, E. J.* Bone regeneration around titanium dental implants in dehisced defect sites. A clinical study. Int J Oral Maxillofac Implants 1992; *7:* 233–245.

[35] *Breine, U., Brånemark, P.-I.* Reconstruction of alveolar jaw bone. An experimental and clinical study of immediate and performed autologous bone grafts in combination with osseointegrated implants. Scand J Plast Reconstr Surg 1981; *14:* 23–48.

[36] *Weidenreich, F.* Über die pneumatischen Nebenräume des Kopfes. Ein Beitrag zur Kenntnis des Bauprinzips der Knochen, des Schädels und des Körpers. (Knochenstudien: II. Teil) Z Anat Entw-Gesch 1924; *72:* 55–93.

[37] *Wood, R. M., Moore, D. L.* Grafting of the maxillary sinus with intraorally harvested autogenous bone prior to implant placement. Int J Oral Maxillofac Implants 1988; *3:* 209–214.

[38] *Lekholm, U., Zarb, G. A.* Patient selection and preparation. In: *Brånemark, P.-I., Zarb, G. A., Albrektsson, T.* (eds). Tissue – Integrated Prostheses. pp. 199–209. Chicago: Quintessence, 1985.

Part 4

Prosthetic aspects of implant-supported prostheses

I. E. Naert

There are often a number of possible solutions for the treatment of a particular patient. Oral implants may be suggested as an alternative, sometimes the only one, for those patients previously destined for conventional prosthodontic treatment (see Chapter 1). Treatment planning and the prosthetic aspects of the rehabilitation of the complete and partially edentulous patient as well as the single tooth replacement by means of oral implants will be considered below. Before the prosthodontic procedure is explained, the different prosthetic designs will be discussed.

Prosthetic designs

For the completely edentulous jaw, four prosthetic designs may be distinguished;

(1) the (fixed) ceramo-metal prosthesis (Fig. 1);
(2) the fixed hybrid prosthesis (Fig. 2);
(3) the removable (detachable) hybrid prosthesis (Fig. 3a and b);
(4) the resilient overdenture (Fig. 4a and b).

Three main factors will determine the choice of design: bone morphology and intermaxillary relationships, the patient's psychological profile and his/her financial situation (Fig. 5).

Bone morphology and intermaxillary relationships

The degree of jaw bone resorption and the subsequent changes in intermaxillary relationship should be considered in connection with the chosen prosthetic design. The degree of jaw bone resorption determines whether teeth, or teeth and hard and/or soft tissues have to be replaced. In the former case, the fixed prosthodontic protocol is followed, involving porcelain fused to metal superstructures (ceramo-metal prosthesis) (Fig. 1). For those patients with moderate to severe resorption, the removable prosthodontic protocol is used. This means that stock tray teeth, in acrylic or porcelain, are attached to the superstructure with pink acrylic resin, thus replacing the lost bone and soft tissues (fixed hybrid prosthesis) (Fig. 2).

For a number of reasons, the use of a removable hybrid prosthesis/detachable prosthesis (Fig. 3a and b) in the maxilla may have advantages over a fixed prosthesis. In such cases there are a sufficient number of implants to support a fixed prosthesis, but owing to the location of the implants, as dictated by anatomical landmarks and/or the intermaxillary relationship, aesthetics,

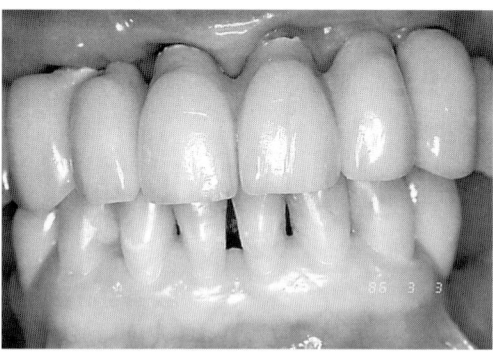

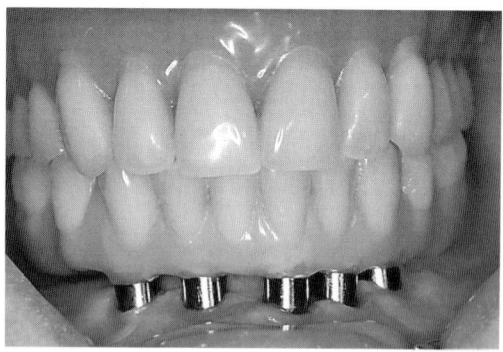

Fig. 1. Ceramo-metal full prosthesis in the maxilla. Limited jaw resorption necessitated the replacement of lost teeth only. The fixed prosthodontic protocol was followed.

Fig. 2. Fixed hybrid full prosthesis in the mandible. Moderate to advanced jaw resorption necessitated the replacement of teeth and bone tissue. The removable prosthodontic protocol was followed.

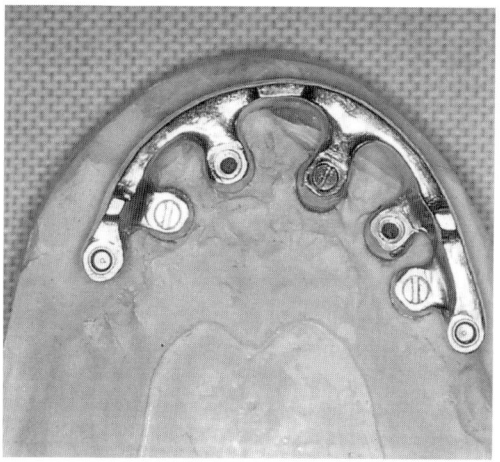

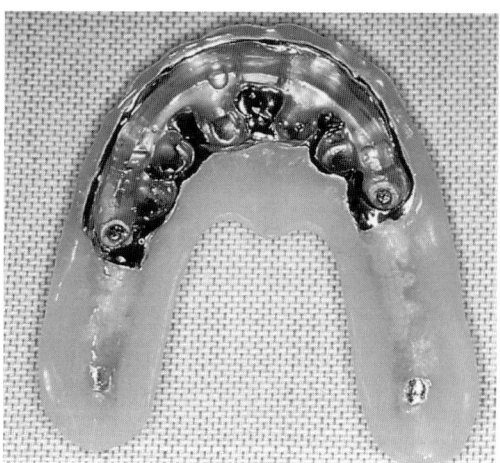

Fig. 3. Removable hybrid full prosthesis in the maxilla. Owing to advanced jaw resorption and an unfavourable intermaxillary relationship, the implants were installed far distal to the anterior teeth. (a) The implants are rigidly connected with a primary cast substructure. (b) By means of a second suprastructure (inner side view), aesthetic, phonetic and prophylactic requirements can better be fulfilled.

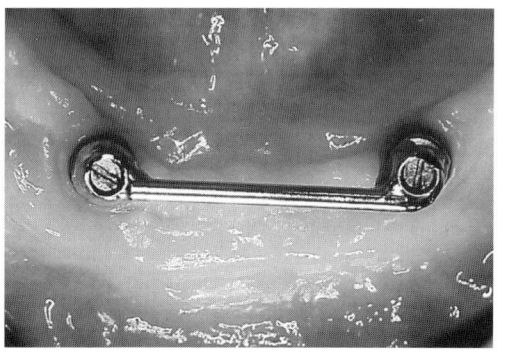

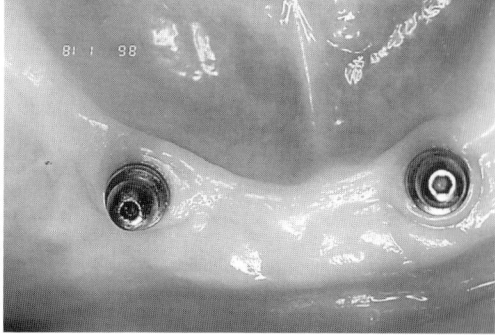

Fig. 4. Two interconnected (a: bar attachment) and two freestanding (b: ball attachment) implants for the stabilization of a resilient mandibular overdenture. Posteriorly, the denture is completely supported by the mucosa. The main advantage of the resilient overdenture is financial.

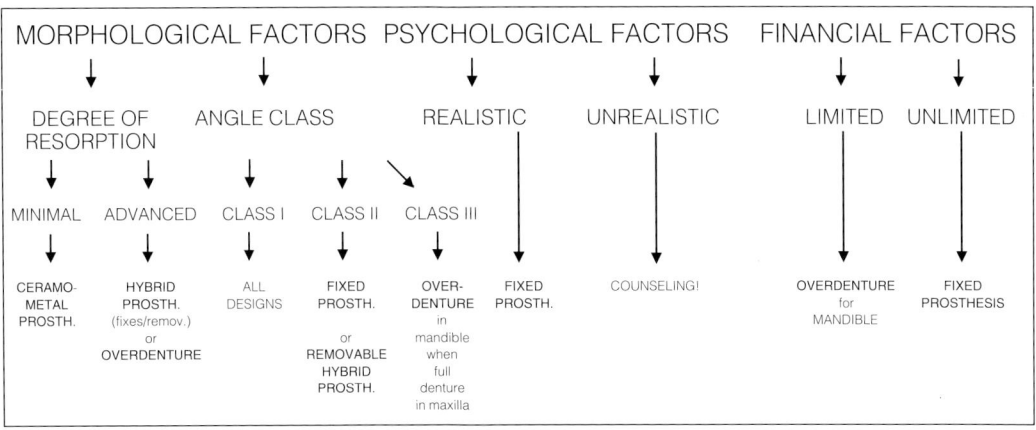

Fig. 5. For the edentulous jaw, the prosthetic design will mainly depend on three factors: jaw bone morphology, the patient's psychologycal status and financial possibilities.

phonetics and oral maintenance may be improved by a removable appliance. In this design it is imperative to connect all implants rigidly by means of a cast rigid primary substructure, in order to distribute the occlusal forces evenly. The length of the "extension" part of the secondary suprastructure should not exceed that of a fixed hybrid prosthesis; this will prevent overloading of the implants. However, a supplementary tooth can be added for aesthetic reasons, but in infraocclusion with the opposing teeth. Some congenital abnormalities such as cleft palate, and surgical defects such as a hemi-maxillectomy, can usually be obturated best with removable dentures. In the presence of an Angle Class II relationship, retrusion of the mandible, the use of a resilient mandibular overdenture (Fig. 4a and b) is contraindicated. Indeed, a resilient overdenture will always tend to hinge around the anterior (imaginary) bar connecting the implants, especially during anterior biting. This will lead to instability of the overdenture during function. When an Angle Class III relationship exists

in a completely edentulous patient, the use of a mandibular fixed implant-supported prosthesis against a complete maxillary denture will tend to focus all the forces onto the anterior maxillary area. This will lead to an unstable maxillary denture and increased resorption in the anterior area.

It is evident that for both the abovementioned intermaxillary relationships, orthognathic surgery may solve the problem much better. However, not every patient may be willing to undergo this kind of surgery.

Psychology of the patient

Psychological assessment will determine whether the prosthesis should be fixed or removable. It is generally accepted that the fixed prosthesis is the treatment of choice for the replacement of missing teeth whenever possible. However, for cosmetic as well as financial reasons, the removable prosthesis may be indicated. One should then try to determine why the patient is

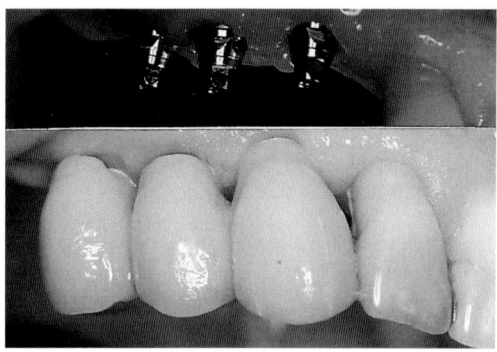

Fig. 6.   Three-unit ceramo-metal partial prosthesis on three implants in the right maxilla. A cantilever prosthesis or a removable partial denture may thus be avoided.

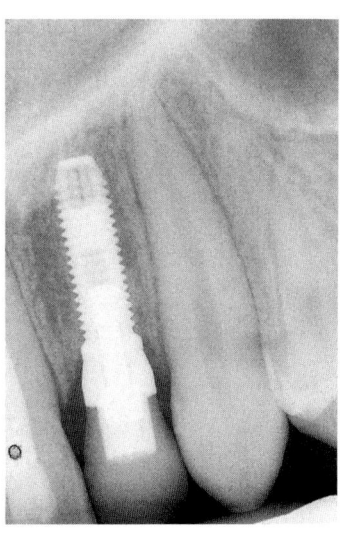

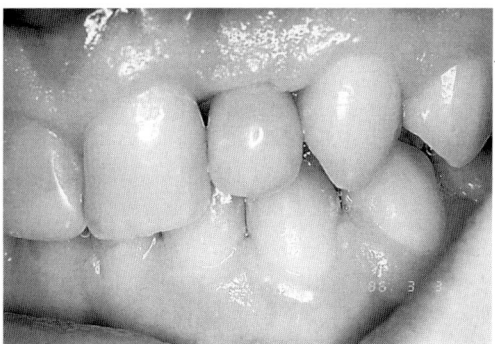

Fig. 7. (a) Single tooth replacement as a substitute for a lost maxillary left lateral incisor in an intact dentition.

(b) Radiograph taken 2 years after loading.

seeking treatment. Is it because of an inability to wear a removable denture, or is the patient looking for greater stability in his/her denture? If the former, then a removable prosthesis is contraindicated and the patient must accept higher cost and; in some instances; some cosmetic compromise or supplementary surgical correction (augmentation, osteotomy, etc.). In the latter case, the patient may have worn a denture for years; but because jaw resorption has progressed, denture stability is compromised. Such patients may be

helped by the installation of two implants, to increase the retention and stability of the denture. Patients with unrealistic demands are referred to other disciplines for personal help (e.g. psychiatry).

Financial considerations

As mentioned previously, the fixed prosthesis is the treatment of choice for most patients. However, because of financial limitations many patients cannot afford these prostheses, especially in countries where the social security system does not cover such treatments. Solutions involving fewer implants may lower the cost. The minimum number of implants which can be installed in the completely edentulous mandible to retain a prosthesis, is two. For elderly patients who have worn a full denture for years, but who complain of instability and lack of retention of their mandibular denture, the installation of two implants and a resilient overdenture is a good alternative to the fixed prosthesis[1-3]. However; patients should be warned that the resorption of the alveolar crest will continue under the mucosa-borne saddles[4]. In younger patients (<45 years), therefore, a resilient overdenture is contraindicated and a fixed prosthesis should be recommended. The resilient overdenture on two implants functions very well in the mandible, but not, at present, in the maxilla. The higher implant failure rate[5] and increased marginal bone loss around the implants[1] contraindicate the use of the resilient overdenture on two implants in the maxilla.

Also, the difference in cost between a full ceramo-metal prosthesis and a hybrid prosthesis may be considerable and, as mentioned earlier, the choice will depend mainly on morphological factors.

In the partially edentulous patient, the ceramo-metal prosthesis (Fig. 6) and the single tooth restoration (Fig. 7a and b) may be distinguished. The (removable) hybrid partial prosthesis may also be indicated (Fig. 8a, 1–2).

In the partially edentulous jaw, the design of choice will be the ceramo-metal prosthesis (Fig. 6) because, as a rule, only teeth will need to be replaced, owing to the reduced resorption in these patients. The disadvantages of acrylic–composite resin veneers are: repeated fracture, especially of the centric cusps, excessive wear and colour instability, leading to unacceptable aesthetics. The rationale for using resin instead of porcelain as occlusal veneering material on implant prostheses is to dampen the occlusal peak forces[6-8] by means of the softer resin teeth. However, *Ismail* and coworkers[9], found no difference in damping characteristics between gold, resin and porcelain when the crown dimensions simulated the clinical situation. Their recommendations were to make the choice between the different materials on the basis of aesthetics and functional requirements. In a clinical follow-up study[10], there was no difference in either the implant failure rate or in marginal bone loss, between prostheses surfaced with resin or porcelain, for up to 2 years. In the prostheses surfaced with resin, a high fracture rate (20%) was noticed compared with the porcelain-surfaced prostheses (0%). The fixed hybrid partial prosthesis is of limited use nowadays. Local alveolar defects should always be considered for correction before or in conjunction with the installation of implants (Fig. 8b, 1–4). Bone correction (membrane technique, bone split technique, grafting technique, etc.) as well as soft tissue correction techniques (flap procedures, tissue expansion, soft tissue inlay, gingivoplasty, etc.) are indicated (see Chapters 5.3 and 11), to improve the aesthetics as well as the load transfer towards the long axis of the implants. This is identical to the standard fixed prosthodontic procedure in which alveolar defects should be corrected surgically to provide optimal aesthetics at the pontic site. The location of the implants in the partially dentate jaw is just as critical as in the edentulous situation with minor resorption of the alveolar crest; single tooth replacement is a great challenge in terms of achieving optimal cosmetic results.

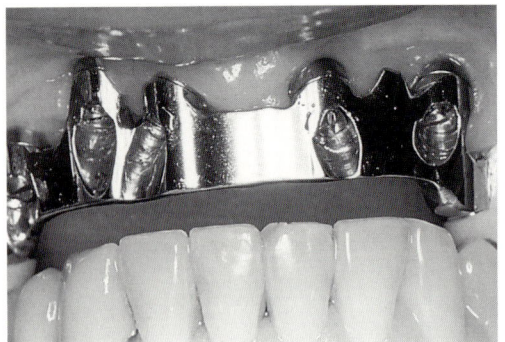

Fig. 8a1

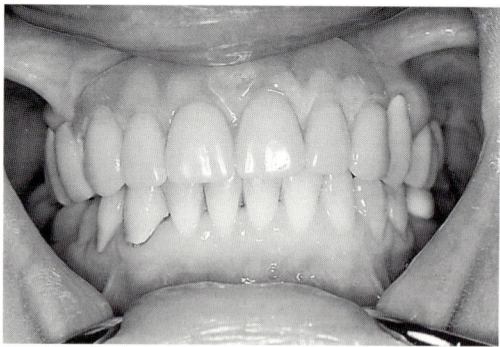

Fig. 8a2

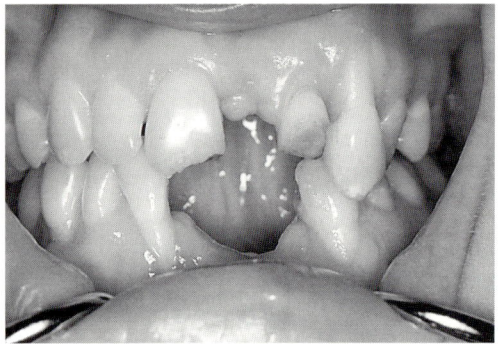

Fig. 8b1

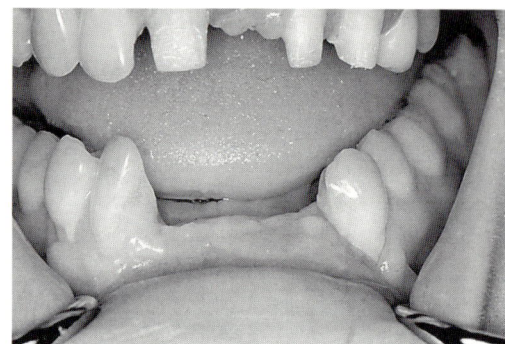

Fig. 8b2

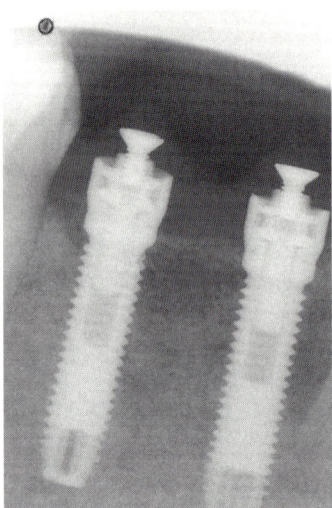

Fig. b3

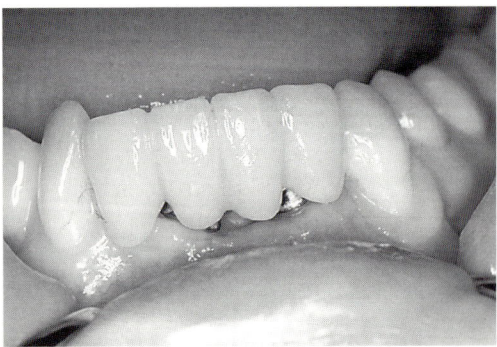

Fig. b4

Fig. 8. Hybrid partial prosthesis (removable). Owing to advanced partial jaw resorption, the hybrid partial prosthesis was used (a 1) Casted primary substructure. (a 2) Situation with the prosthesis in place. The ceramo-metal prosthesis (b) may be indicated also, provided there has been a correction of the alveolar crest . Before treatment (b 1). Extraction of the 42 and grafting procedure coincided with implant installation (b 2- 3). After prosthesis installation (b 4).

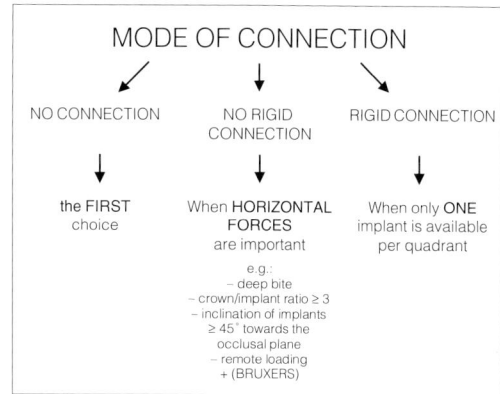

Fig. 9. Protocol for connecting teeth with implants.

Connection between teeth and implants

Three modes of connection may be used in the partially edentulous patient; unconnected or freestanding, not rigidly connected and rigidly connected (Fig. 9). The choice depends on the need to distribute the occlusal forces, not only on the implants but on the teeth as well. Because of differences in mobility characteristics between teeth and implants (see Chapter 7) the primary choice will always be the freestanding or unconnected prosthesis. As it is well-known that six, five or even four implants can support a ten-unit prosthesis over a long period[11], it is tempting to argue that two to three implants should be able to support a three- to five-unit partial prosthesis equally well. Several studies support this argument[12–14]. However, some factors differ compared with the complete implant-supported prosthesis. In the complete fixed prosthesis, there is always cross-arch stabilization, in that the implants on the right are rigidly connected with those on the left side. In the partially edentulous patient this cross-arch connection is absent. This means that freestanding implants in the

partially edentulous arch are more prone to remote or non-axial loading and eventually to overloading, leading to implant loss, severe marginal bone loss and implant fatigue fracture.

Situations involving particular risk are:

(1) Patients with deep bites, where articulation takes place only in the region of the implant-supported prosthesis;
(2) When the distance between occlusal plane and bone level is more than three times the length of the osseointegrated implant;
(3) When the artificial teeth are remote from the long axis of the implants;
(4) When the angle of the implants deviates significantly from the perpendicular to the occlusal plane (Fig. 10).

The risk of implant failure and complications increases when patients exhibit parafunctional activity (heavy bruxism). In all of these situations, connecting implants to teeth to achieve cross-arch stabilization, may help to distribute the occlusal forces. However, a prerequisite for this is that the mobility of the teeth is within normal physiological limits (<0.1 mm). When teeth exhibit greater mobility, this should be reduced to approximately the same level as that of the im-

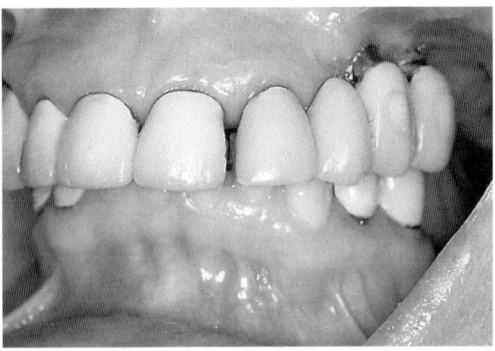

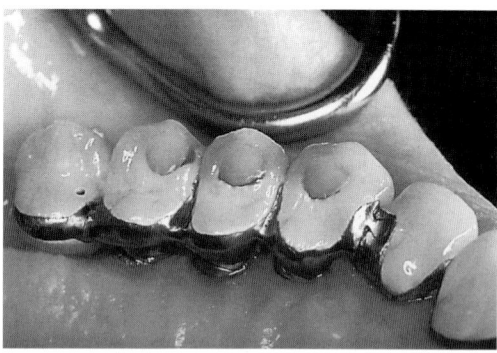

Fig. 10. Partial prosthesis on two inclined implants (23 and 24), 45° towards the loading direction, in the presence of a deep bite. This lead to implant fatigue fracture, 3 years after loading.

Fig. 11. Partially edentulous patient with a deep bite, articulation contact on the working side only of the implant-supported prosthesis, besides parafunctional activity. A non-rigid connector (between 13 and 12, the 12 was part of an 8-unit bridge) is applied to splint teeth with implants ($n = 3$) in a cross-arch connection to improve the load distribution.

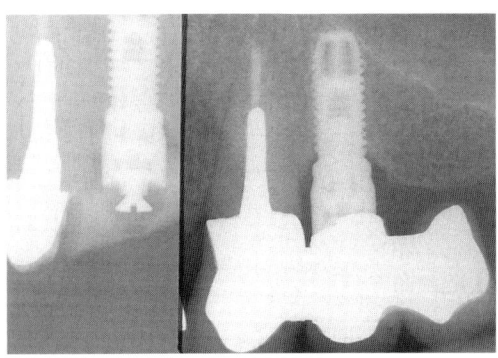

Fig. 12. The installation of only one implant distal to the canine necessitated splinting the implant with the canine. A rigid connection prevents slippage of the male in the female part, especially in combination with a cantilever pontic in this 3-unit prosthesis. (a) Situation at abutment connection and (b) 3 years after bridge installation.

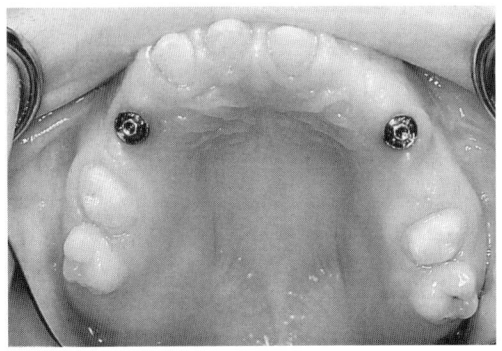

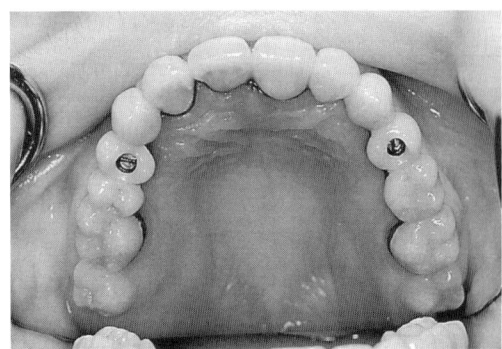

Fig. 13. Two implants were installed in the left (25) and right (15) maxilla of a young girl with partial agenesis (a) to improve the retention of a 12-unit ceramo-metal bridge (b). To simplify the construction; a rigid connection was aimed for. Luting with a temporary luting cement enables periodical removal of the bridge to control implant stability.

plants. This may be achieved by splinting several teeth in a rigid prosthesis. It should be borne in mind that a two-stage implant system should not be considered as completely rigid[15]; because of the two junctions in the system: first, the junction between implant and the abutment, and secondly; the junction between the abutment and the prosthesis. These screwed junctions allow a certain degree of flexibility of the implant system during function or parafunction. This may help the stress distribution when teeth are connected with implants. Other systems have a built-in "artificial ligament", made of plastic, e.g. the intra-mobile element of the IMZ implant, which is intended to simulate the periodontal ligament (see Chapter 5, Part 2). Although the damping characteristics of these devices have been demonstrated[16], their beneficial effects have not yet been demonstrated in terms of fewer implant failures, less marginal bone loss or fewer mechanical problems. However, the passive fit of a screwed framework on implants with a plastic material between implant and prosthesis instead of metal–metal contact is evidently less critical in the former case. To what extent (30 µm or 100 µm) the misfit between implants and prosthesis framework can be tolerated before implant failure or complications occur, is not yet known.

Whenever a cross-arch connection is indicated, for example when increased horizontal forces are expected, a non-rigid connector (1 degree of freedom, in the vertical plane) may suffice to distribute the occlusal forces between teeth and implants (Fig. 11). A rigid connection (0 degrees of freedom) is indicated when only one implant can be incorporated in the prosthesis (Fig. 12) or when a number of implants are distributed between several teeth. In the former situation, if a non-rigid connection is used, there is a greater risk that, due to

wear, the male part will separate from the female part, creating severe distortion, especially when a cantilever pontic is part of the prosthesis[10, 15, 17]. When a few implants are located between several teeth, for ease of construction, which usually also implies increased longevity, rigid connection is advocated (Fig. 13a and b).

In summary, there should be no connection when there is no obvious reason for it. Connection will be considered in those situations where increased horizontal forces may be expected or when only one implant is present per quadrant.

Luting versus screw superstructures

A screwed superstructure has the great advantage that the prosthesis can easily be removed, whenever necessary, without damage to the implants or the superstructure. This is necessary to investigate individual implant stability (see Chapter 9). When the prosthesis is permanently fixed to several implants; it is not possible to check individual implant stability. Clinically, mobility measurements are still the only means of confirming the presence or absence of osseointegration. The slightest mobility in an individual implant implies a failure. It means that direct bone apposition is absent and that fibrous tissue has intervened, which may lead eventually to infection.

Retrievability is also helpful when repairs are necessary to the prosthesis. When screwed superstructures are used, the path of insertion is not as critical as for luted superstructures, in which all the "cores" need to be exactly parallel. However, screwed superstructures require optimal passive fit on the implants. For aesthetic reasons, the access holes for the set screws must be located on the occlusal surface.

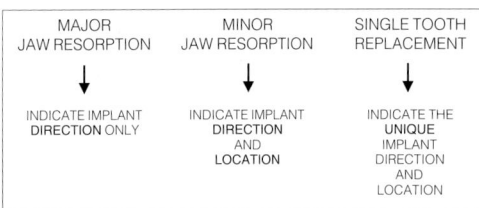

Fig. 14. Surgical stent requirements depending on the resorption status and prosthetic design.

The disadvantages of the screwed superstructures are the advantages of the luted superstructures. By luting the superstructure, the location of the access holes for the set screws becomes unimportant. The tolerance of fit, at least within limits, <40 µm, is greater for luted than for screwed structures. Small fitting errors of the superstructure may be "corrected" by the thickness of the luting cement. However, unless a temporary luting cement is used, the superstructure is no longer retrievable. This implies that control of stability of each implant is no longer possible. Although a small cement gap does no harm to the implants (metal–metal) when the prosthesis–implant junction is located supragingivally, in the case of subgingival junctions, luted superstructures become much more critical. Indeed, as with teeth, subgingival margins lead to gingivitis and eventually to periodontitis. However, the relationship between gingivitis and "peri-implantitis" is not completely understood and still controversial. Unless more data become available, it is best only to bring the crown margins subgingivally when the patient requires it for aesthetic reasons. Machined and highly polished screwed joints should be used here.

Prosthodontic procedures

The prosthodontic procedures may be divided into two stages: the preliminary and the final treatment stage.

Pretreatment planning

Once the decision has been made to treat the patient by means of oral implant, following careful patient selection (see Chapter 4), it is up to the prosthodontist to plan where and in what direction the implants should ideally be placed. The most important factors which will dictate these positions are the available bone volume, the willingness of the patient to have the bone volume augmented by surgical procedures and the aesthetic expectations of the patient. This means that the patient should be examined by both the surgeon and the prosthodontist. The surgeon will use radiographic techniques to assess the height and width of the jaw bone and anatomical landmarks in relation to the number, length, position and angle of the implants. The prosthodontist will gain supplementary information by mounting study casts at the correct vertical dimension in the articulator. This will help in judging the maximum length of the lever arms in the final restoration. For more difficult cases, teeth should be set up in the laboratory and eventually tried in the patient. This procedure is especially useful for all maxillary edentulous patients and for the restoration of a partially edentulous maxillary anterior region. Here, a decision should be made to improve the location, direction and number of planned implants by means of "non-standard" surgical procedures (see Chapter 5.3). To transfer the information from the tooth set-up to the mouth, a

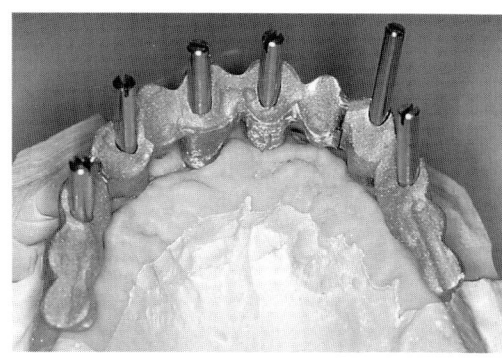

Fig. 15. Cast framework for a ceramo-metal fixed full prosthesis in a maxilla showing limited resorption. The location and direction of the implants is vital in achieving optimal results. The implants are just beneath each tooth and the long axes of the implants are perpendicular towards the occlusal plane. By using a surgical stent and pre-operative planning, optimal installation of the implants is guaranteed.

surgical stent/template/index/indicator is made. The purpose of the stent will differ; depending on alveolar crest height, the status of the jaw, whether the patient is completely or partially edentulous or whether it is a case of single tooth replacement (Fig. 14).

Surgical stent for the completely edentulous jaw

When the alveolar crest is only minimally resorbed, as is usual following recent tooth extraction, only the missing teeth need replacement. This also means that the abutments will pierce through the mucosa at a distance of one tooth length from the occlusal plane. This situation will force the surgeon to install every implant just beneath and in the long axis of the artificial teeth on the prosthesis. This will improve the aesthetic, phonetic and prophylactic characteristics of the final restoration (Fig. 15). The surgical stent should indicate the location as well as the direction of every implant in the jaw bone. This can be done by making a transparent acrylic template, indicating the buccal surfaces of every tooth. It can also be done using an acrylic template indicating the long axis of the implant by means of guiding holes for the drills, or by adding acrylic posts on the template.

Several designs are possible; depending on the preference of the surgeon.

When the jaw bone shows a moderate to advanced resorption, not only teeth but also hard and soft tissues have to be replaced. The abutment will now pierce the mucosa at a greater distance from the occlusal plane. The location of the implants will no longer be critical in relation to the end result for aesthetics, phonetics and ease of maintenance. The implants should be installed, as perpendicular as possible to the occlusal plane. This avoids perforation of the access holes for the set screws of the prosthesis in the buccal surfaces and allows the most favourable load transfer to the implants. The surgeon has complete freedom mesio-distally to install the implants. This means that the posterior implants on both sides should be positioned as far distally as possible, taking into account the anatomical landmarks, the anterior sinus wall for the maxilla, and the mental foramen for the mandible. This approach leads to maximal spread of the implants, decreasing the cantilever lengths and the compression loads on the distal implants and the tension loads on the more mesial implants. The prosthodontist will, therefore, provide the surgeon with a stent which only indicates the direction of the implants, not the location (Fig. 16). The surgical stent for the edentu-

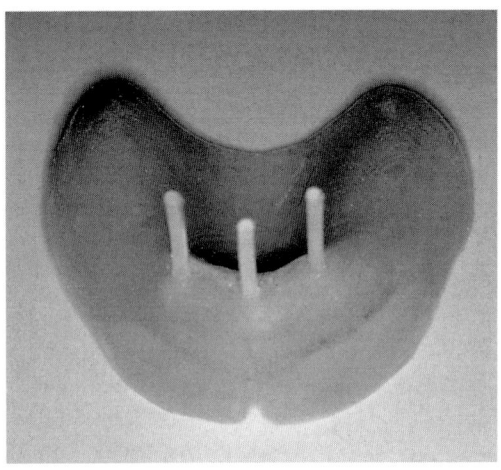

Fig. 16. Typical surgical stent, indicating only the direction of the implants. This is used when moderate to advanced jaw resorption has occurred, so that the mesiodistal location of the implants with respect to the long axis of the teeth is no longer important.

lous jaw will be made on the opposite jaw, preventing contamination of the surgical site during implant installation. However, a prerequisite for the correct use of this stent is that the surgeon should use it when the mandible is in centric relation at the appropriate vertical dimension. During surgery; the chosen sites are marked directly on the alveolar crest by means of a round bur, after the mucoperiosteal flap has been raised. Perforation of the mucoperiosteal flap just above the implant sites is better avoided, if one wishes to follow the principle of hermetic closure of the soft tissues after implantation.

Surgical stent for the partially edentulous jaw

In the partially edentulous jaw the alveolar crest usually shows only limited resorption. This means that the abutment will pierce the mucosa at one crown length from the occlusal plane. Again, *direction* and *location* of

the implants are critical to achieve optimal results (Fig. 17 a, b and c). However, in contrast to the edentulous jaw, the surgical stent is made on the same jaw, supported by the remaining teeth. Here the surgeon should neither guide the mandible into centric relation, nor should he be aware of the vertical dimension.

Surgical stent for single tooth replacement.

Because of its location, usually in the anterior maxilla, the single tooth replacement is the most critical in terms of the aesthetic result. The surgeon has little if any freedom to choose the position of the implant. The surgical stent completely dictates the direction and location of the implant. A stent with one drilling hole gives the prosthodontist the assurance that the patient will get what he or she was promised in terms of optimal aesthetics (Fig. 18). When luted crowns are used, there is a greater degree of freedom

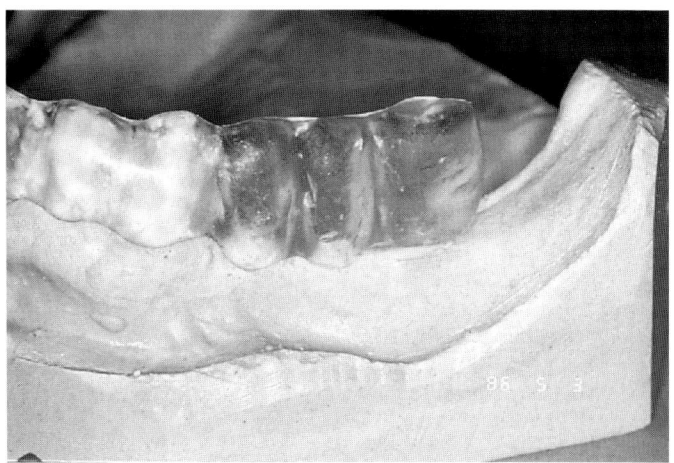

Fig. 17. a) Partial surgical stent indicating the buccal tooth surfaces;

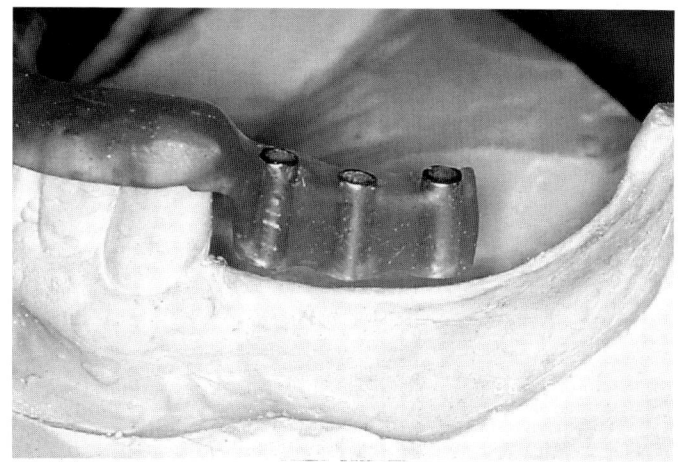

b) Position and direction of the implants are indicated by means of drill holes;

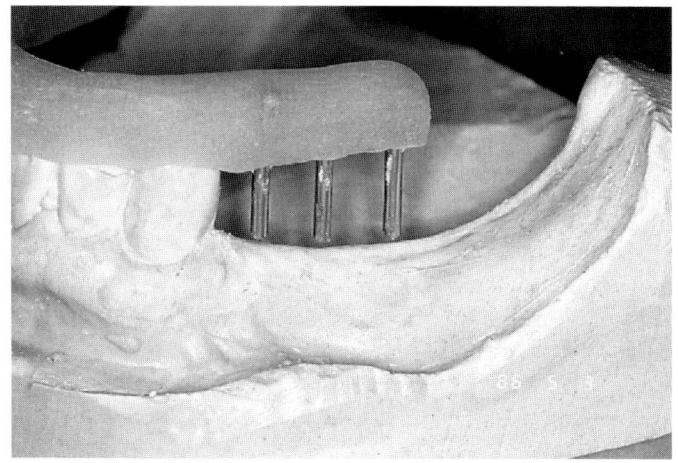

c) A third possibility is to use posts fixed on a resin template.

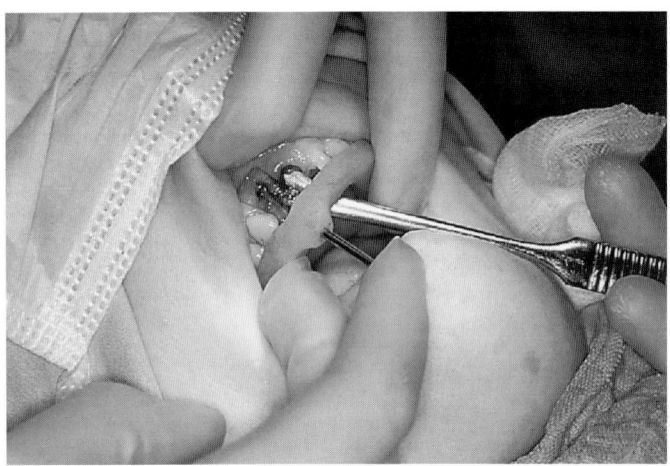

Fig. 18. Control with a surgical stent for single tooth replacement, in which only one position is dictated during implant installation. This guarantees optimal aesthetics for the patient.

in the buccolingual direction, as compared to screwed crowns.

It must be understood that, using the surgical stent; the ideal sites are indicated with respect to the final restoration. Even when one assesses the jaw bone anatomy and quality prior to surgery with tomograms or CT scans, small deviations of location and especially of direction from the surgical stent still occur. The surgeon must always bear in mind that implants should be installed to direct occlusal forces favourably under all conditions of loading and with regard to achieving optimal aesthetic, phonetic and hygiene results. However, implants should not be installed in positions dictated by the stent, if such positions would seriously compromise the survival of an implant. Bone quality is, at present, still best evaluated during surgery.

Whenever pronounced deviations from the surgical stent exist, they should be recognized in advance and discussed with the patient. Alternative surgical procedures such as bone augmentation techniques, sinus lifting and grafting procedures, dis-

placement of the mandibular nerve bundle etc., as well as prosthetic alternatives such as split-cast/double superstructures or removable/detachable hybrid prostheses, may then be considered.

Final treatment stage

The objective of this phase of treatment is the fabrication of an absolutely passive fitting prosthesis with the highest rigidity, together with acceptable occlusion and articulation, allowing optimal oral maintenance and optimal aesthetics. A distinction should be made between the provisional and final prosthesis.

Provisional prostheses

Once the abutments are connected to the implants, the implants are connected by means of a rigid superstructure. This may be a provisional one or the final one. The fabrication of a provisional prosthesis has several advantages:

(1) Allows control of the osseointegration when the implants are loaded;
(2) Allows optimal soft tissue healing;
(3) Allows optimal abutment choice (for two-phase systems);
(4) Allows bone remodelling without peak force transmission in the early healing phase;
(5) Allows prediction of speech patterns and aesthetics.

One of the most important advantages of using provisional prostheses is the possibility of clinically judging osseointegration (the absence of mobility, confirmed by the absence of radiolucency around the implant). It should be borne in mind that the presence of a radiolucent area only confirms the lack of osseointegration; the converse is not true. Thus, following abutment connection, absence of mobility of the implant is the only criterion the clinician has to judge the osseointegration of that implant. However, at this stage the implants have not yet been loaded, so that a definite judgement cannot be made. Loading the implants by means of a rigid provisional prosthesis for some months gives the clinician a better indication as to whether the implants will remain osseointegrated even after loading. Therefore, provisional prostheses should be considered in all cases in the maxilla and in the post-foraminal area in the mandible. The chance that an implant in the inter-foraminal area will be lost after abutment connection is rather small (see Chapter 5.2). The requirements for provisional prostheses are the same as those for the final prostheses; optimal passive fit, maximum rigidity and ease of oral maintenance. The provisional prosthesis is made of acrylic resin and, if necessary, is fibre-reinforced. All factors that may contribute to axial loading of the "osseointegrating" implants should be considered (e.g. avoid cantilever pontics and try to distribute the occlusal forces over all present implants). Another advantage when working with provisional prostheses is the possibility of optimal healing of the soft tissues around the abutments. If the implant system is of the two-phase design, the "healing" abutment may be changed to the appropriate one, before taking the final impression. A shorter abutment may improve aesthetics or increase the intermaxillary space, the angulated abutment may compensate for the implant inclination. Before the final prosthodontic phase is undertaken; the provisional prosthesis is an excellent aid in reassessing the planned prosthetic design. If the patient cannot become accustomed to a fixed prosthesis because of phonetics or aesthetics, or if the design is difficult for the patient to maintain, the use of a removable hybrid prosthesis may be the final choice for that patient. This situation may occur in the completely edentulous maxilla, when the location of the implants deviates considerably from the original tooth positions. The use of a provisional prosthesis is always an advantage, never a waste of time and energy.

Prosthodontic procedures

The prosthetic treatment for implant-supported prostheses is shown in Fig. 19.

Modifications of the prosthesis after surgery

Ten to twelve days after implant installation, the existing denture or an interim prosthesis is lined with a soft lining material (tissue conditioner) if the patient is wearing a removable denture or the fixed prosthesis is temporarily luted to the neighbouring teeth. The removable denture is liberally relieved above the implant site, and prosthesis flanges are shortened if they are too long.

PROSTHODONTIC TREATMENT SEQUENCE

I. Modifications after surgery	II. Fabrication of provisional prosthesis	III. Fabrication of final prosthesis
– Interim prosthesis lined with **tissue conditioner** after implant installation – Fixed temporary prosthesis adapted on abutment teeth.	– Except for interforaminal area	– Preliminary impression taking – Final impression taking – Jaw relations' registration – Try-in tooth set-up – Try-in of casted framework – Prosthesis insertion – Recall

Fig. 19. Flow chart indicating the prosthetic treatment for the implant-supported prosthesis.

In the intial healing period, the soft tissue lining is frequently replaced. In partial edentulism the advantage of the teeth is that a fixed prosthesis "protects", the implants from external forces (functional as well as parafunctional). Therefore, a fixed prosthesis should always be considered whenever abutment teeth have to been prepared to carry fixed prostheses, before implants are installed. When the patient is wearing removable dentures (complete or partial) he/she is warned to leave the prosthesis out as much as possible. This will protect the implants from unnecessary loading. During the healing period, the patient is told to take a soft diet for the same reason. It is the responsibility of the practitioner who makes the prosthesis to monitor the patient carefully during the healing period. Following the initial healing period, two-monthly recall appointments to check further soft tissue healing, would not be excessive.

The provisional prosthesis

Following abutment connection, the objective is to splint all implants as soon as possible with a provisional prosthesis, except those in the inter-foraminal area, where the final prosthesis can be applied immediately.

The final prosthesis

Preliminary impression taking. One week after abutment connection, the preliminary impression should be taken. This involves fabrication of the custom tray, which yields more information, not only about the implant site but also about other anatomical features.

Final impression taking. Depending on the system used, the custom tray will be closed or open above the implant site. Systems in which the impression copings are fixed into the impression material and unscrewed before removing the impression are recommended (pick-up technique). Accuracy is further improved when the impression is taken using impression plaster. Before the impression is poured, abutment replicas are attached onto the impression copings. After the plaster has set and the impression removed from the master model, the abutment replicas are in exactly the same position, relative to each other, as they were in the mouth.

Registration of jaw relations

This is identical to standard prosthodontic protocol. In completely edentulous patients, considerable stability is gained for the wax occlusion rims by means of the implants.

Try-in of the teeth

Before modelling the wax pattern for the metal framework; a set up of acrylic teeth is done in wax on a trial denture base and eventually tried in the patient. The try-in should, as far as possible, be identical in form and shape to the final restoration. Only in this way can the patient really evaluate the end result. When satisfied, the wax-up of the framework can start. The two main objectives should be: optimal passive fit and maximum rigidity, together with hygienic design. The two objectives are very closely related to each other. Maximum rigidity, which will distribute the occlusal forces optimally, makes a passive fitting framework imperative. Indeed, especially with screwing devices, a misfit of one part of the prosthesis will lead to high stress concentrations in the implant in that area[18, 19]. This will cause marginal bone loss around the crestal part of the implant, possible implant component fracture and, eventually, loss of osseointegration.

Try-in of the cast framework

After casting the framework in a non-corroding metal alloy, the try-in is performed on the patient. This is the most critical and difficult phase and is one of the main keys to success or failure of the implants. A misfit will sooner or later result in biological or mechanical implant failure.

Up to now there are no data available to indicate the tolerance of misfit before failure becomes clinically significant; nor is there a clinical device which may quantify the magnitude of that misfit. Therefore, the only means of judging framework fit are meticulous visual inspection of the abutment–prosthesis junction, the absence of strain felt by the patient when screwing the prosthesis and clinical experience. When the junction is open on one or more sites, the framework has to be sectioned, plaster-indexed in the mouth and soldered. Finally, the prosthetic teeth are attached with heat-cured acrylic resin to the framework or, in the case of a ceramo-metal prosthesis, porcelain is fused onto the metal structure. Maintenance of the passive fit after fusing of the porcelain is not assured. Special measures have to be taken, but these will not be discussed further here.

Handing over the prosthesis

Again a meticulous check of the passive fit is carried out, together with the occlusion and articulation; according to standard prosthodontic protocol[20]. The patient is instructed in the maintenance of the device and abutment areas and he/she warned not to "overdo it" when chewing, especially for edentulous patients who will need a learning period to get used to their "third dentition".

Recall

The patient is enrolled in a recall program. One week after installation of the prosthesis a check-up is carried out for oral maintenance, occlusion and articulation and, in the case of a screwed prosthesis, all set screws are retightened. Depending on the needs of the patient, he/she should be seen every 6 to 12 months (see Chapter 9).

References

[1] Naert, I., Ouirynen, M., Theuniers, G., van Steenberghe, D. Prosthetic aspects of osseointegrated fixtures supporting overdentures. A 4-year report. J Prosthet Dent 1991; 65: 671–680.

[2] Mericske-Stern, R. Clinical evaluation of overdenture restorations supported by osseointegrated titanium implants. Int J Oral Maxillofac Implants 1990; 5: 375–383.

[3] Kirsch, A., Ackerman, K.-L. The IMZ osseointegrated implants system. Dent Clin North Am 1989; 33: 733–761.

[4] Jacobs, R., Schotte, A., van Steenberghe, D., Quirynen, M., Naert, I. Posterior jaw bone resorption in osseointegrated implant supported overdentures. Clin Oral Impl Res 1992; 3: 63–70.

[5] Engquist, B., Bergendal, T., Kallus, T., Linden, U. A retrospective multicenter evaluation of osseointegrated implants supporting overdentures. Int J Oral Maxillofac Implants 1988; 3: 129–134.

[6] Skalak, R. Aspects of biomechanical considerations. In: Tissue-integrated prostheses. Osseointegration in clinical dentistry. pp. 117–128. Berlin: Quintessence Publ Co Inc, 1985

[7] Brunski, J. B. Biomaterials and biomechanics in dental implant design. Int J Oral Maxillofac Implants 1988; 3: 85–97.

[8] Brunski, J. B. Biomechanics of oral implants: Future research direction. J Dent Educ 1988; 52: 775–787.

[9] Ismail, Y., Kukunas, S., Pipho, D., Ibiary, W. Comparative study of various occlusal materials for implant prosthodontics. J Dent Res (special issue/abstract) 1989; 68: 962.

[10] Naert, I., Quirynen, M., van Steenberghe, D., Darius, P. A six-year prosthodontic study of 509 consecutively inserted implants for the treatment of partial edentulism. J Prosthet Dent 1992; 67: 236–245.

[11] Adell, R., Eriksson, B., Lekholm, U., Brånemark, P.-I., Jemt, T. A long-term follow-up study of osseointegrated implants in the treatment of totally edentulous jaws. Int J Oral Maxillofac Implants 1990; 5: 347–359.

[12] Jemt, T., Lekholm, U., Adell, R. Osseointegrated implants in the treatment of partially edentulous patients: A preliminary study on 876 consecutively placed implants. Int J Oral Maxillofac Implants 1989; 4: 211–217.

[13] van Steenberghe, D., Lekholm, U., Bolender, C., Folmer, T., Henry, P., Herrmann, I., Higuchi, K., Laney, W., Lindén, U., Åstrand. The applicability of osseointegrated oral implants in the rehabilitation of partial edentulism: A prospective multicenter study on 558 fixtures. Int J Oral Maxillofac Implants 1990; 5: 272–281.

[14] Quirynen, M., Naert, I., van Steenberghe, D., Dekeyser, C., Callens, A. Periodontal aspects of osseointegrated fixtures supporting a partial bridge. An up to 6-years retrospective study. J Clin Periodontol 1992; 19: 118–126.

[15] Rangert, B., Gunne, J., Sullivan, D. Y. Mechanical aspects of a Brånemark implant connected to a natural tooth: An in vitro study. Int J Oral Maxillofac Implants 1991; 6: 177–186.

[16] Chapman, R. J., Kirsch, A. Variations in occlusal forces with a resilient internal shock absorber. Int J Oral Maxillofac Implants 1990; 5: 369–374.

[17] Sullivan, D. Prosthetic considerations for the utilization of osseointegrated fixtures in the partially edentulous arch. Int J Oral Maxillofac Implants 1986; 1: 39–45.

[18] Davis, D. M., Zarb, G. A., Chao, Y.-L. Studies of the frameworks for the osseointegrated prostheses: Part I. The effect of varying the number of supporting abutments. Int J Oral Maxillofac Implants 1988; 3: 197–201.

[19] Jemt, T., Carlsson, L., Boss, A., Jörneus, L. In vivo load measurements on osseointegrated implants supporting fixed or removable prostheses: A comparative study. Int J Oral Maxillofac Implants 1991; 6: 413–417.

[20] Beyron, H. Occlusion; point of significance in planning restorative procedures. J Prosthet Dent 1973; 30: 641–652.

Chapter 6

Oral motor function and phonetics in patients with implant-supported prostheses

S. Karlsson and G. E. Carlsson

Oral rehabilitation with a removable denture, both in partially and completely edentulous patients, implies a perturbation to the oral cavity. Most patients are satisfied with their conventional removable dentures, but there are a number of individuals with varying degrees of adaptation difficulties to removable dentures, and a smaller number who are unable to accept removable prostheses at all. This might be explained by a combination of ageing, anatomical, physiological and psychological factors[1-3].

Many functional tests are used to demonstrate impaired oral motor function (mastication, speech, etc.) in patients with removable dentures in comparison with dentate controls[4-6]. This may in part be attributed to a reduction in denture retention and stability. Associated speech problems are also common, at any rate during the first period after prosthetic rehabilitation. Even with optimal prostheses, many oral functions appear impaired[6]. A removable prosthesis may cause adaptive problems more often than a fixed one and some studies indicate that the problems are frequent (Table I).

Table I. Adaptation difficulties with removable dentures[1, 2]

Removable partial dentures	
Dentures no longer used	31%
Complete denture wearers	
Can chew only soft or mashed food (2% of the 70-year-old edentulous subjects did not wear any dentures, 11% did not wear lower dentures)	29%
Cannot chew all types of food	24%
Assess their chewing ability as poor	9%

It is, therefore, easy to understand why the concept of osseointegrated implants for retention of oral prostheses as a treatment modality has stimulated great interest, in both patients and dentists.[7-10]

Oral rehabilitation with osseointegrated implants in the edentulous patient appears at first to offer only advantages and benefits, but there are some functional drawbacks. In this chapter, some of these problems are described and the background data are examined. This will hopefully contribute to an understanding of a hypothetical problem and will possibly suggest means to meet clinical situations which may be encountered.

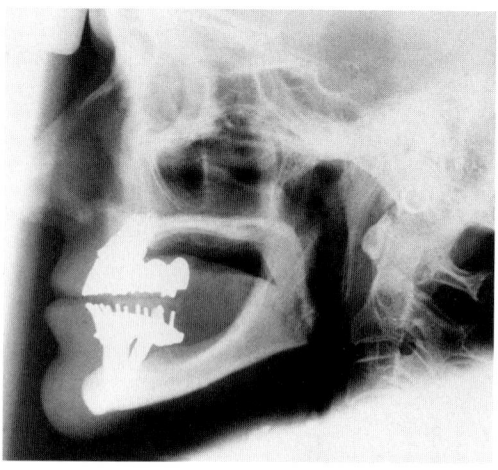

Fig. 1. Lateral radiogram indicating the anterior location of the implant-supported fixed prostheses.

Oral motor function in the edentulous patient before and after rehabilitation

Patients' own assessment of oral functions

A useful way of subjectively evaluating the functional capacity of the masticatory system is by means of questionnaires. In this way it is possible to determine the patients' own judgement of their oral function. Several studies using such questionnaires have shown convincingly that the great majority of patients treated with oral implants were very satisfied with their oral functions. This was true for the first cross-sectional studies[11], as well as for the longitudinal investigations which directly compared pretreatment and post-treatment evaluations[10, 12–15]. Positive answers were received concerning the stability of the implant prostheses as well as improved chewing ability. Before treatment, many patients had to avoid certain foods, while only

a few had difficulty chewing a limited number of foods after treatment. These reports are in agreement with the fact that practically all treated patients perceived the implant prosthesis as an integrated part of themselves. In a long-term survey of treated patients, several remarks were noted in response to questions on the aesthetic results of the prostheses, acceptance of small shortcomings of details and phonetic adaptation. Initial phonetic problems were, however, reported by 60% of the patients. Problems were mainly associated with the "s"-sound, but these were of short duration and disappeared after an adaptation period[16, 17]. The overall assessment of the rehabilitation was extremely favourable. The subjective experience of functional improvement also appeared to affect the patient in a broader sense, e.g. increased self-confidence and improved general psychological outlook[9].

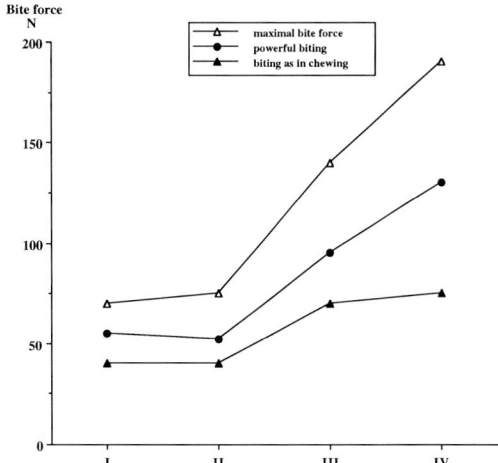

Fig. 2. Bite force at three force levels at four sessions:[10]
I = old complete dentures; II = new complete dentures; III = two months after insertion of a mandibular implant-supported fixed denture; IV = three years after insertion.

Craniomandibular dysfunction (CMD)

Compared with the natural tooth and its periodontal ligament, an implant has a rigid interface with the jaw bone and the occlusal contact pattern has often been given an anterior location with shortened dental arches (Fig. 1). These facts have elicited some concern regarding overload on components of the masticatory system, particularly the temporomandibular joint, and subsequent CMD. However, patients treated with osseointegrated implant-retained prostheses have, in general, reported few and mainly mild symptoms of CMD, and this has been confirmed by clinical examination. Pre-existing symptoms appeared to diminish after treatment, an observation that was also noted in a longitudinal study, involving reports from both before and after implant treatment[13]. Consequently, temporomandibular joints and masticatory muscles seem to respond favourably to this treatment, suggesting a good prognosis for stomatognathic function.

Bite force

Bite force measurements have been used as an indicator of masticatory function. In healthy subjects with an almost complete natural dentition, the maximum bite force in the molar region averages 300 to 500 N, although there is great individual variation[4, 5]. Removable dentures are associated with a reduction in bite force, which is most pronounced in complete denture wearers; conventional fixed partial dentures (FPD) are not usually associated with such a reduction. In a longitudinal study of complete denture wearers who received osseointegrated implant-supported FPDs, the initial mean maximum bite force was 69 N[10]. Two months after insertion of the implant prosthesis, bite force had increased by 85% and after 3 years the mean force was almost three times the pretreatment value (Fig. 2). These results have been confirmed by other studies[18]. By using a technique that employed six strain gauge transducers, the investigators were able to simultaneously analyse the force pattern in different regions of the jaws during biting and chewing[19]. The

125

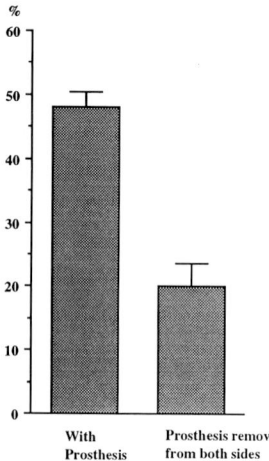

Fig. 3. Masticatory efficiency before and after removing a partial implant-supported fixed denture in the mandibular lateral segments[21].

functional forces recorded for the implant-supported FPD patients were close to those in patients with FPDs on natural teeth.

Chewing efficiency

The most commonly used direct measurement of the capacity to reduce a test food to small particles is the so-called comminution test. This is usually based on a system of sieves[4], and the results of such tests have shown that chewing efficiency decreases as the natural occlusion deteriorates, and is worse for subjects with complete dentures. In patients treated with implant-supported FPDs, the chewing efficiency was comparable with that in a matched control group with a natural dentition[20]. Neither the chewing rate nor the chewing time differed.

In a longitudinal study of completely edentulous patients, optimal conventional treatment with complete dentures did not significantly change the chewing efficiency[6]. Two months after insertion of an FPD supported by implants in the mandible, a significant improvement had occurred,

and this was substantiated by a reduction in both chewing time and the number of chewing strokes necessary for comminuting the test food. Three years after treatment, the index value for chewing efficiency was even better, indicating a gradual improvement through adaptation.

When partially edentulous patients are treated with an implant FPD in the lateral segments of the jaw, chewing efficiency is again improved[21]. A dramatic decrease of chewing efficiency occurred immediately after the partial implant-supported teeth were removed, which emphasizes the importance of those teeth in mastication (Fig. 3).

Consequently, patients treated with implant-supported FPDs seem to benefit from this type of rehabilitation, which increases their ability to comminute food.

Chewing pattern

The obvious improvement of the patients' subjective assessment of masticatory func-

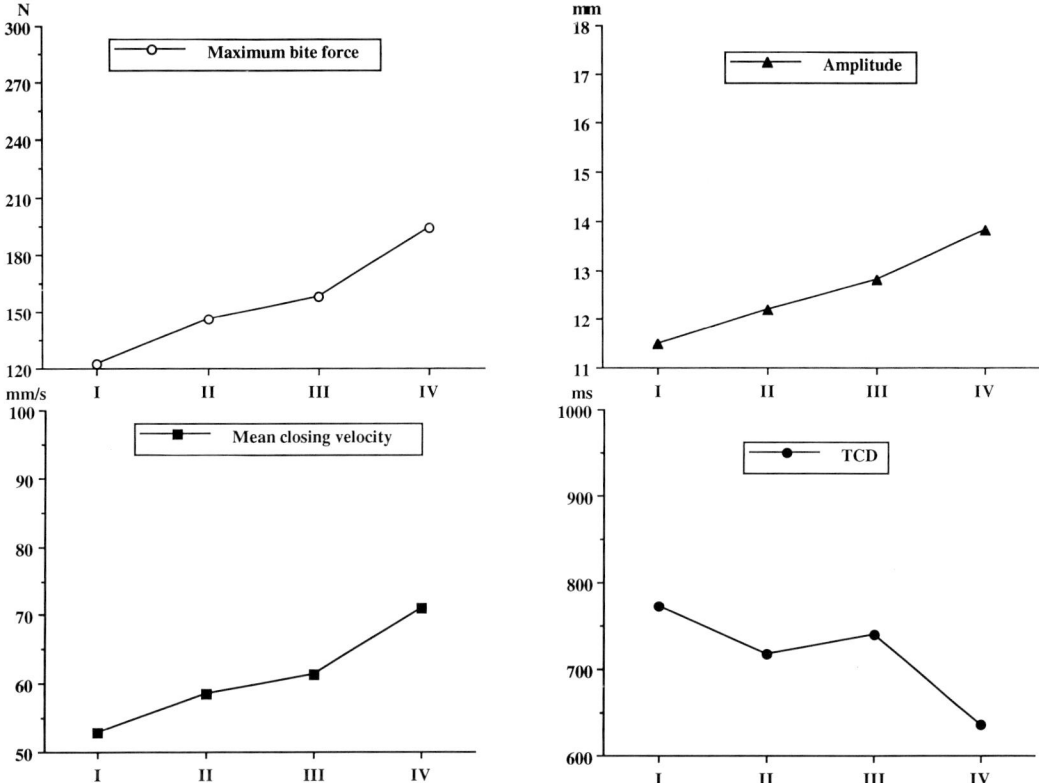

Fig. 4. Maximum bite force, mandibular velocity, opening displacement and masticatory cycle duration at four sessions[18]: I = at insertion of an implant-supported fixed denture; II = 1 week post insertion; III = 3 months post insertion; IV = 1 year post insertion.

tion following treatment with an implant-supported FPD could also be verified in objective changes in chewing patterns[22]. This has been studied in complete denture wearers by recording masticatory mandibular movements both before and during a 10-year period, following treatment with an implant FPD in the lower jaw[23]. The general chewing pattern was not changed to any great extent after insertion of an implant FPD. However, some of the studied parameters of oral motor function did show apparent alteration, with a registered increase in mandibular velocity and displace-ment (Fig. 4). The total duration of the masticatory cycle tended to decrease, with a significant reduction in the slow closing phase. This was interpreted as a consequence of the stabilization of the prostheses and improved sensory feedback following the insertion of the mandibular implant FPD. Handling the bolus should also be facilitated and will further contribute to improved oral function after rehabilitation. The placement of a maxillary osseointegrated FPD in some patients did not appear to significant-ly further change the variables investigated. This could imply that, even if the mechanism

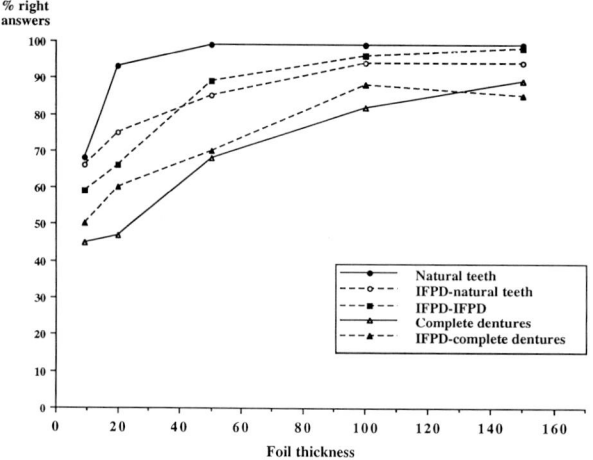

% right answers

Foil thickness

Legend:
- Natural teeth
- IFPD-natural teeth
- IFPD-IFPD
- Complete dentures
- IFPD-complete dentures

Fig. 5. Correct answers when testing occlusal tactile sensitivity in subjects with a natural dentition, complete dentures and implant-supported fixed dentures[30].

is multifactorial, rehabilitation of the edentulous mandible is more significant than of the maxilla, in terms of improvements in masticatory function.

Neurophysiological functions

The periodontal receptors are thought to be important for the afferent encoding of mechanical stimulation of the teeth and consequent oral motor function. Information from these receptors are also used for the moment-to-moment modulation of different motor programs needed for the control of mastication. After the loss of teeth, most of these receptors are lacking and could perhaps be compensated for by other receptor systems. These patients are therefore neurophysiologically interesting and a number of studies have investigated their neuromotor system. Different studies have looked at

(1) Reflex activity;
(2) Muscular function;
(3) Occlusal tactile sensitivity.

Reflex activity and sensorimotor function

The jaw unloading reflex is of great importance clinically. When biting on a hard object, large isometric forces are developed and if this reflex is lacking, the teeth will crash together when the object breaks. The reflex is therefore thought to be part of a protective mechanism, to arrest sudden and unexpected mandibular closing movements, damaging to the stomatognathic system. The origin of this reflex has not, so far, been fully elucidated, but possible receptors are thought to be situated in the periodontal ligaments, joints, tendons, and muscles. Edentulous patients with implant FPDs lack the periodontal receptors. Partly as a consequence of this, it has been proposed that acrylic resin should be used for the occluding surfaces in implant-supported FPDs, to provide the system with shock protection between the implant and the occluding surfaces and thereby avoid overload of the implant/bone interface[24].

Periodontal ligament receptors are believed to be mainly responsible for the generation of the silent period. Experimental[25–27] results showed that the subjects with an implant FPD in both jaws failed to elicit such a reflex. Important information provided by the periodontal receptors, includes the direction and point of application of a load to an individual tooth [27, 28]. There is no convincing evidence that this fact creates a drawback for motor control in patients with implant FPDs.

Muscular function

Muscular function in subjects with a natural dentition and those rehabilitated with implant-supported prostheses has been compared by means of electromyography (EMG)[11, 29]. The mean voltage amplitude was practically the same in both tested groups, both for postural activity and during biting and swallowing.

Occlusal tactile sensitivity

In order to assess tactile function, foils of varying thickness are placed between opposing teeth. The test subject is instructed to report if he or she can feel the foil or judge whether it is thicker or thinner than a previous one.

To clarify the role of the periodontal receptors in this discrimination task, a number of studies have been carried out, comparing edentulous, dentate and partially dentate subjects[30, 31]. Subjects with a natural dentition showed the lowest interocclusal detection and discrimination thresholds, at the 20 μm level. Corresponding values for patients with osseointegrated FPDs in one or both jaws were two to three times this value; for complete denture wearers; the value was five times higher, in the order of 100 μm (Fig. 5). It may be concluded that partial or complete lack of periodontal

receptors is partly compensated for by other receptor organs, and that osseointegrated implant FPD therapy contributes to the restoration of occlusal sensitivity.

An important clinical implication of this is that subjects who are edentulous or have implant-supported FPDs, are less able to detect occlusal discrepancies. It is therefore important that the treating dentist should take extra care when giving the final shape to the occlusion. It has been shown in experimental studies that occlusal interferences as small as 80 μm substantially changed the force distribution in implant-restored dentitions[19, 32, 33]

Oral adaptation

According to current definition, adaptation means "the ability to make something suitable for a new need". Evidently, patients rehabilitated with full-arch osseointegrated implant FPD are lacking mechanosensitive receptors in the periodontal ligament. As mentioned earlier, however, there are indications that other receptor systems will take over and compensate for this[25, 26]. Studies of edentulous patients receiving implant-supported FPDs have indicated that the process of adaptation involves two steps. An early, immediate change of recorded variables and a later, more time-dependent phase[18, 23].

In a study of edentulous patients treated with FPDs on osseointegrated implants[18], masticatory cycle duration and maximum bite force changed significantly during the first week after installation (Fig. 4). This early change might be the result of improved peripheral mechanosensitive input, following restoration with a fixed prosthesis. It could also be a psychological central effect, a subjective feeling of safety with the new fixed prosthesis. In other studies, new complete dentures alone did not have this effect[6]. This, together with improved sensorimotor function following rehabilitation with a fixed prosthesis on implants must be considered to be important for the overall outcome and prognosis.

Minimal changes occurred during a subsequent period of 1 week to 3 months; this might be interpreted as a plateau in the learning or adaptation process. One year later, recordings again showed significant and pronounced changes in certain variables. Mandibular velocity, movement amplitude and bite force had increased[18]. These changes in oral motor function may be the result of learning and adaptive changes of central processes and cortical engrams governing the final motor output.

Phonetics and speech production

A very complex neurophysiological mechanism lies behind the production of speech and a number of oral mechanosensitive receptors are involved in its motor control. All prosthodontic treatment involves clinical procedures which may influence speech performance. Functional studies have shown that about half the edentulous patients who were treated with implant FPDs experienced speech difficulties, mainly during the first weeks after insertion[34]. Similar results have been reported in a 3-year follow-up study of subjects recorded before and after rehabilitation with implant FPDs[17]. From a dental point of view, the "s"-sound is most interesting, since this is mainly influenced by the teeth. The design of the palatal part of the maxillary prosthesis and its incisors are important factors for the articulation of "s". Speech difficulties in connection with prosthodontic treatment may also be related to problems concerning:

(1) The space available for the tongue;
(2) The shape of the palatal surface of the anterior teeth;
(3) The width of the interdental space.

Few studies have investigated speech production in relation to prosthetic rehabilitation, in particular after implant FPD treatment. In a recent study, however, there is convincing evidence of adaptation taking place in a fairly short time[17]. One third of pretreatment patients, wearing a complete denture, reported subjectively deteriorated speech. Immediately after implant FPD treatment, about 60% experienced some problems with speech. At the 3-year follow-up, however, only 5% considered themselves to have any speech problems whatsoever. An interesting finding was that open or closed interdental spaces were not related to speech problems.

In conclusion, according to the studies presented, extensive maxillary oral rehabilitation requires a rather long period of adaptation before values are back to baseline or improved. There is no indication that rehabilitation with a maxillary implant FPD will be accompanied by any definite phonetic problems in comparison with other prosthodontic treatment methods. On the contrary, this therapy may help to meet phonetic functional demands.

Summary

A number of studies have shown that substantial functional improvement results from treatment with an osseointegrated FPD in edentulous patients. The objectives of oral rehabilitation, namely to restore masticatory, phonetic and aesthetic functions are therefore attained. Masticatory function following implant rehabilitation is equal to, or very close to, that found in subjects of the same age with a natural dentition. This improvement is confirmed through patient assessments, clinical examinations, and various clinical experimental studies. The decisive factor appears to be the stability of the FPD supported on firmly osseo-integrated implants, in contrast to complete dentures with their comparatively poor retention and stability. This enables patients to revert to a more normal physiological situation, similar to that seen with natural teeth.

Functional improvement is fundamental to overall recovery, which includes psychosocial reactions and enhanced quality of life. This is frequently reported by patients following implant FPD treatment and has been verified in controlled studies.

References

[1] Carlsson, G. E., Hedegård, B., Koivumaa, K. K. Late results of treatment with partial dentures. An investigation by questionnaire and clinical examination 13 years after treatment. J Oral Rehabil 1976; 3: 267–272.

[2] Österberg, T. Odontologic studies in 70-year-old people in Göteborg (Thesis). Sweden: University of Göteborg, 1981.

[3] Carlsson, G. E. Masticatory efficiency: The effect of age, the loss of teeth and prosthetic rehabilitation. Int Dent J 1984; 34: 93–97.

[4] Carlsson, G. E. Bite force and chewing efficiency. In: Kawamura, Y. (ed.). Frontiers of oral physiology. 1. Physiology of mastication. pp. 265–292. Basel: Karger, 1974.

[5] Bates, J. F., Stafford, G. D., Harrison, A. Masticatory function – a review of the literature. III. Masticatory performances and efficiency. J Oral Rehabil 1976; 3: 57–67.

[6] Lindqvist, L. W., Carlsson, G. E., Hedegård, B. Changes in bite force and chewing efficiency after denture treatment in edentulous patients with denture adaptation difficulties. J Oral Rehabil 1986; 13: 21–29.

[7] Brånemark, P.-I., Hansson, B.-O., Adell, R., Breine, U., Lindström, J., Hallén, O., Öhman, A. Osseointegrated implants in the treatment of the edentulous jaw. Experience from a 10-year period. Stockholm: Almqvist & Wiksell, 1977.

[8] Brånemark, P.-I., Zarb, G. A., Albrektsson, T. Tissue-integrated prostheses. Osseointegration in clinical dentistry. pp. 11–76. Berlin: Quintessence Publishing Co., 1985.

[9] Blomberg, S. Psychological response. In: Brånemark, P.-I., Zarb, G. A., Albrektsson, T. (eds). Tissue-integrated prostheses. Osseointegration in clinical dentistry. pp. 165–174. Berlin: Quintessence Publishing Co., 1985.

[10] Lindqvist, L. W., Carlsson, G. E. Long-term effects on chewing efficiency and bite force of treatment with mandibular fixed prostheses on osseointegrated implants in complete denture wearers. Acta Odontol Scand 1985; 43: 39–45.

[11] Haraldson, T., Carlsson, G. E., Ingervall, B. Functional state, bite force and postural muscle activity in patients with osseointegrated oral implant bridges. Acta Odontol Scand 1979; 37: 195–206.

[12] Lindqvist, L. W. On prosthetic rehabilitation of the edentulous mandible. A longitudinal study of treatment with tissue-integrated fixed prostheses. Swed Dent J 1987; Suppl. 48.

[13] Lundqvist, S., Carlsson, G. E. Maxillary fixed prostheses in osseointegrated dental implants. J Prosthet Dent 1983; 50: 262–267.

[14] Haraldson, T., Zarb, G. A. A 10-year follow-up study of the masticatory system after treatment with osseointegrated implant bridges. Scand J Dent Res 1988; 96: 243–252.

[15] Naert, I., De Clercq, M., Theunier, G., Schepers, E. Overdentures supported by osseointegrated fixtures for edentulous mandibles: a 2.5-year report. Int J Oral Maxillofac Implants 1988; 3: 191–196.

[16] Jemt, T., Carlsson, G. E. Aspects of mastication with bridges on osseointegrated implants. Scand J Dent Res 1986; 94: 66–71.

[17] Lundqvist, S., Haraldson, T., Lindblad, P., Speech in connection with maxillary fixed prostheses on osseointegrated implants: a three-year follow-up study. Clin Oral Implant Res 1992; 3: 176–180.

[18] Book, K., Karlsson, S., Jemt, T. Functional adaptation to full-arch fixed prosthesis supported by osseointegrated implants in the edentulous mandible. Clin Oral Implant Res 1991; 3: 17–21.

[19] Lundgren, D., Laurell, L., Falk, H., Bergendal, T. Occlusal force pattern during mastication in dentitions with mandibular fixed partial dentures supported on osseointegrated implants. J Prosthet Dent 1987; 58: 197–204.

[20] Haraldson, T. Comparisons of chewing patterns in patients with bridges supported on osseointegrated implants and subjects with natural dentitions. Acta Odontol Scand 1983; 41: 203–208.

[21] Tzakis, M., Lindén, B., Jemt, T. Oral function in patients treated with prostheses on Brånemark osseointegrated implants in partially edentulous jaws: A pilot study. Int J Oral Maxillofac Implants 1990; 5: 107–111.

[22] Jemt, T., Stålblad, P.-Å. The effect of chewing movements on changing mandibular complete dentures to osseointegrated overdentures. J Prosthet Dent 1986; 55: 357–361.

[23] Karlsson, S., Jemt, T. Adaptive changes of masticatory movement characteristics after rehabilitation with osseointegrated fixed prostheses in the edentulous jaw. A 10-year follow-up study. Int J Maxillofac Implants 1991; 6: 259–263.

[24] Skalak, R. Biomechanical considerations in osseointegrated prostheses. J Prosthet Dent 1983; 49: 843–848.

[25] Bonte, B., van Steenberghe, D. Masseteric post-stimulus EMG complex following mechanical stimulation of osseointegrated oral implants. J Oral Rehabil 1991; 18: 221–229.

[26] Brodin, P. Fløystrand, F., Ørstavik, J. The masseteric reflex evoked by tooth and denture tapping. J Oral Rehabil 1991; 18: 327–335.

[27] Mühlbradt, L., Ulrich, R., Möhlmann, H., Schmid, H. Mechanoperception of natural teeth versus endosseous implants revealed by magnitude estimation. Int J Oral Maxillofac Implants 1989; 4: 125–130.

[28] Trulsson, M., Johansson, R. S., Olsson, K. Å. Directional sensitivity of human periodontal mechanoreceptive afferents to forces applied to the teeth. J Physiol 1992; 447: 373–389.

[29] Haraldson, T., Ingervall, B. Muscle function during chewing and swallowing in patients with osseointegrated oral implant bridges. An electromyographic study. Acta Odontol Scand 1979; 37: 207–216.

[30] Lundqvist, S., Haraldson, T. Occlusal perception of thickness in patients with bridges on osseointegrated oral implants. Scand J Dent Res 1984; 92: 88–92.

[31] Jacobs, R., van Steenberghe, D. Comparative evaluation of the oral tactile function by means of teeth or implant-supported prostheses. Clin Oral Implant Res 1991; 2: 75–80.

[32] Carr, A. B., Laney, W. R. Maximum occlusal force levels in patients with osseointegrated oral implant prostheses and patients with complete dentures. Int J Oral Maxillofac Implants 1987; 2: 101–108.

[33] Falk, H. On occlusal forces in dentitions with implant-supported fixed cantilever prostheses. Swed Dent J 1990, Suppl. 69.

[34] Jemt, T. Failures and complications in 391 consecutively inserted fixed prostheses supported by Brånemark implants in edentulous jaws. Int J Oral Maxillofac Implants 1991; 6: 270–275.

Chapter 7

Biomechanics of osseointegration and dental prostheses

J. B. Brunski and R. Skalak

Osseointegration has been defined as "the direct structural and functional connection between ordered living bone and the surface of a load-carrying implant"[1]. The fixation of oral implants to bone by means of osseointegration has allowed highly predictable, long-term functional performance of implant-supported bridgework, especially in the fully edentulous patient and increasingly in the partially edentulous patient. A full understanding of the success and limitations of osseointegration in both types of patients involves biomechanics.

There is an increasing appreciation of the vital role that biomechanics plays in the performance of oral implants. The aim of this chapter is to provide some basic principles that will allow a clinician to formulate a biomechanically valid treatment plan. However, at this point in the history of oral implantology, the clinician should realize that we do not know enough to provide absolute biomechanical rules that will guarantee success of all implants in all situations. There are always differences between patients in terms of key factors such as the amount of available bone, bone quality, number of missing teeth, masticatory habits, etc. Consequently, our limited goal is to inform the clinician about how one can apply biomechanical concepts to devise a rational treatment plan

and to assess its limitations. To examine the key biomechanical questions, one must begin with an analysis of the distribution of biting forces to implants. Related topics, such as stress transfer to surrounding tissues and interrelationships between bone biology and mechanical loading are major subjects, deserving a separate discussion. Some additional references provide more detail[2, 3].

The relevance of biomechanics to the oral implant problem may be appreciated by analogy to a much simpler, more commonplace problem, namely hanging a picture on a wall using some type of fastener. In picture-hanging, the main factors to consider are the weight of the picture and frame, and the selection of a fastener to hang the picture frame to the wall. The weight of the frame is easy to measure or estimate. Also, the direction in which the weight acts is obvious: it acts downwards due to gravity. However, selecting a fastener to attach the picture to the wall isn't so easy. One fastener may work in certain situations but not others. A decision about which fastener to use will depend on the nature of the wall, since not all walls have the same properties. In fact, as everyone knows, there are different types of fasteners, screws, nails, anchors, etc., for different types of walls.

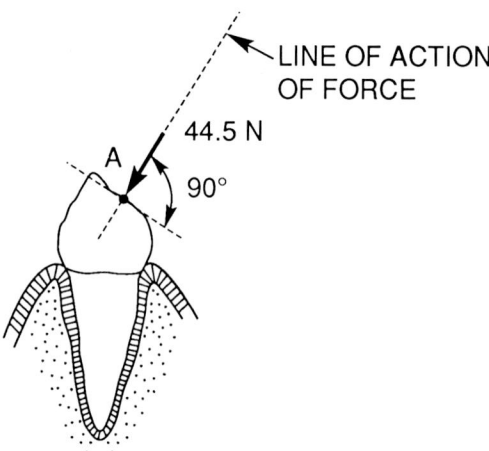

LINE OF ACTION OF FORCE

44.5 N

A

90°

Fig. 1. Diagram of a tooth loaded by a 44.5 N force acting along a line of action which is perpendicular to the surface of the tooth at A and not parallel to the long axis of the tooth.

Although the analogy between picture-hanging and oral implantology is imperfect, it does draw attention to the mechanical basis of both problems. The biomechanics of dental prostheses may be regarded in analogous stages. First, there is a need to know the loadings (bite forces) exerted on the prosthesis. Secondly, one needs to know the distribution of the applied forces to the implants and teeth supporting the prosthesis. (As will be seen, this distribution depends strongly on the number of abutments, their location/orientation in the arch and the properties of the abutments and surrounding bone.) Thirdly, the force on each implant must be delivered safely to the bony tissues over the long term, which in turn depends a great deal on the shape and size of the implant. In all of this, the aim of biomechanical analysis is to forestall failure of any part of the system, including the prosthesis, the supporting implants and the biological tissues.

There are a number of questions to be considered. First, if a clinician wants to place oral implants so that a certain type of full-arch prosthesis will be supported, how many implants should be installed and exactly how should they be spaced and oriented for the best results? Should the clinician simply place as many implants as possible in the available bone? Again, if a clinician wants to design a partial denture to be supported partly by teeth and partly by implants, is this a good idea? While the current state of knowledge makes it difficult to answer either of these questions absolutely, the goal of this chapter is to provide a set of biomechanical principles on which to base an analysis.

Forces on prostheses, supporting implants and natural teeth

Forces and force components

During mastication, the jaw muscles act in concert to close the jaws, causing the teeth to shred and crush food into manageable particles that can be swallowed. There are

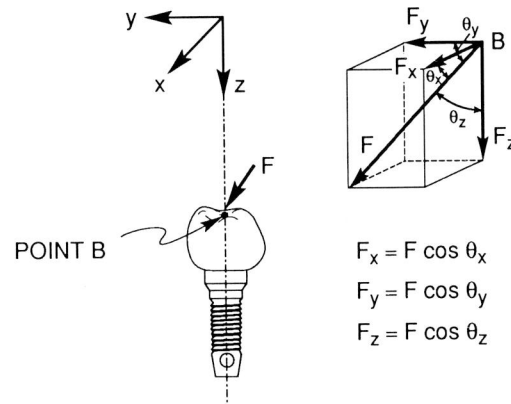

$F_x = F \cos \theta_x$

$F_y = F \cos \theta_y$

$F_z = F \cos \theta_z$

Fig. 2. A force F acting on the pontic at point B may be resolved into components directed along the x-, y- and z-axes.

a number of factors that determine the forces on the teeth or implants during this process. In order to discuss these factors using the correct terminology, it is appropriate to review a few basic concepts of mechanics, including the definitions of force and force components.

Defined loosely as a push or a pull, a force is typically measured in the units of pounds (lb, in the U.S. Customary System of Units), or Newtons (N, in the Système International d'Unités, or SI system). (The conversion is 1 lb = 4.448 N.) In general, force is a vector quantity. A vector has both magnitude and direction. In contrast, a scalar quantity, such as temperature, humidity, or density, is characterized by its magnitude alone; there is no need to specify directionality to define the quantity further. While the size (magnitude) of a force may be expressed in units of lb or N, the magnitude alone is not a complete description of the force because, in general, it is also important to know the direction in which the force is acting. For example, a 10 lb force acting downwards on a tooth does not have the same effect as a 10 lb force acting sideways.

There are various ways of denoting vectors in mechanics. For the purposes of illustrating forces in diagrams, a force vector is represented as an arrow, with the arrow's length being proportional to the magnitude (size) of the vector force, and the arrow's direction showing the direction in which the force acts. This direction is called the line of action. Furthermore, in dealing with forces and how they affect structures – in particular teeth, implants and bridgework – it is also important to specify the point of action of the vector. For example, Fig. 1 shows a force vector of magnitude 44.5 N (10 lb) acting along a line of action which is perpendicular to the surface of a tooth at point A. Vectors are usually written in bold face ($\mathbf{F}$) or with an arrow over the symbol ($\bar{F}$). To indicate the magnitude of the vector, one simply writes F.

Another important concept is the idea of resolving a force vector into components. For example, in Fig. 2, assume that a 44.5 N force arises due to point-contact between a small spherical particle of food and the surface of a tooth crown during chewing. Suppose that the crown is supported by a

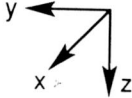

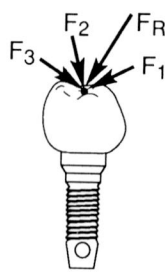

Fig. 3. The vector sum of three forces F_1, F_2 and F_3 is the resultant force F_R, whose magnitude and direction are found using an analysis based on adding the components of the forces (see text).

single underlying implant. Note that in Fig. 2 the force does not act in a direction parallel to the axis of the implant. Suppose that the force here acts at point B which is along the centre line of the implant. The question arises: What part of the applied force acts parallel to, and what part acts perpendicular to, the axis of the implant? This question is relevant in the case where an implant or some part of it, might fracture if the perpendicular component becomes too large. The way to analyse this problem is to resolve the force vector into components along the directions of interest. To do this, a coordinate system with x-, y- and z-axes at right angles to one another (a so-called Cartesian coordinate system) and with the z-axis parallel to the long axis of the implant is selected (Fig. 2). Then, by considering the angles that the force vector makes with the three coordinate axes, it is possible to resolve the force into its three components: F_z (acting along the z-axis) and "sidewise" components F_x, F_y (acting along the x- and y-axes). The components of **F** are defined and computed by the following equations:

$$F_x = F \cos \theta_x \qquad (1)$$
$$F_y = F \cos \theta_y \qquad (2)$$
$$F_z = F \cos \theta_z \qquad (3)$$

In these equations, **F** is the scalar magnitude of the force, equal to 44.5 N in our example. θ_x, θ_y and θ_z are the angles between the force vector and the x-, y- and z-axes, respectively. A useful relationship exists between the magnitude of the force (F) and the values of its three components, F_x, F_y and F_z:

$$F = \sqrt{F_x^2 + F_y^2 + F_z^2} \qquad (4)$$

Equation (4) follows from the definitions, Eqs. (1, 2, 3), and a known geometric relationship among the three angles, namely:

$$\cos^2\theta_x + \cos^2\theta_y + \cos^2\theta_z = 1 \qquad (5)$$

To illustrate this using some numbers, if it is known that the angles θ_x and θ_y are 60° and 70°, respectively, then θ_z can be computed to be about 37° from Eq. (5). Then, the values of F_x, F_y and F_z can be calculated from Eqs (1, 2, 3) to be 22.3, 15.2, 35.4 N, respectively, when **F** = 44.5 N.

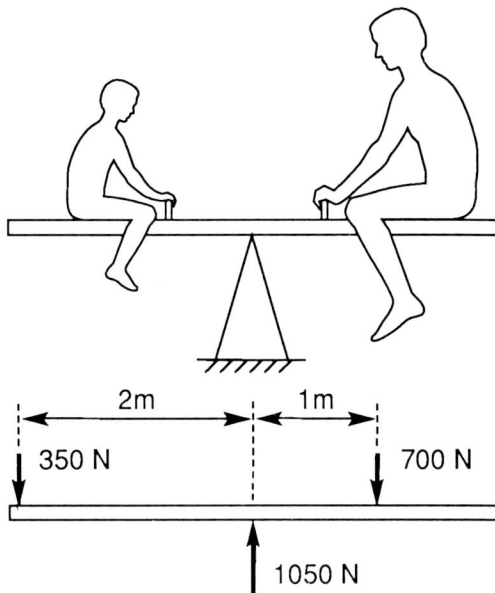

Fig. 4. Static equilibrium, as illustrated by an elementary see-saw: when the system is balanced (no motion), the sum of the moments about the fulcrum is zero, and the sum of the forces is also zero.

As suggested by the above analysis, the intuitive notion that chewing forces always act parallel to the long axes of teeth and implants is, at best, an oversimplification and is, in general, false; there can be lateral as well as vertical force components acting at the same time on a tooth or implant. While it is probably true that the largest component is usually the vertical component, this is not necessarily the only component present. During grinding of the teeth, the lateral component may be the largest.

Another useful concept from mechanics is the idea of vector addition. If more than one force is acting on some object, then the resultant force is the vectorial sum of all the forces acting on the body. For example, in Fig. 2, the force **F** may be regarded as the resultant of combining three mutually perpendicular vectors whose respective magnitudes are F_x, F_y and F_z. Similarly, in Fig. 3, the force resultant F_R is formed from a vector sum of $F_1 + F_2 + F_3$. The way to find the magnitude of the resultant of several forces acting on a body is to follow three steps:

(1) Resolve each force to be added into its three components;

(2) Sum like components by Eqs (1, 2, 3) i.e. add all the F_x's of the forces, etc. This sum is the x-component of the resultant force. Compute F_y and F_z similarly;

(3) Compute the square root of the sum of the squares of the component sums by Eq. (4). This gives the magnitude of the resultant force, F_R.

To find information about the line of action of this resultant, we compute the angles that the resultant force makes with the three coordinate axes θ_x, θ_y and θ_z using Eqs (1, 2, 3), $\cos^{-1} \theta_x = F_x/F_R$, etc.

Finally, another necessary concept from mechanics is the idea of a moment, or torque. Basically, a moment or torque is an action which tends to rotate a body. The dimensions of a moment are force times

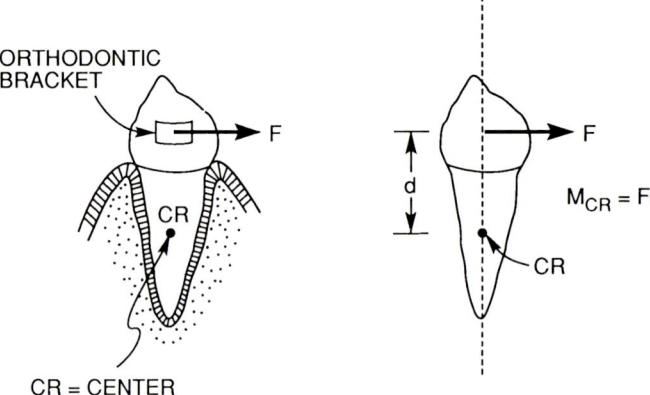

Fig. 5. Example of a moment being produced on a tooth during orthodontic treatment: when the force is applied at the level of the crown, the moment about the centre of rotation (point CR) is Fd.

distance; typical units are N·m or N·cm in the SI system, and lb·ft or oz·in in the English system. For example, in using a screwdriver, the hand supplies a spinning action to the handle of the screwdriver to turn it. The effect of forces applied by the hand is to produce a moment, or torque, about the axis of the screwdriver. Another elementary example of a moment comes about when two children of different weight balance one another on a see-saw. The see-saw is balanced because there are equal moments about the center point of the see-saw (Fig. 4). In a more clinically relevant example, an orthodontic force applied to the crown of a natural tooth produces a moment about its center of rotation which in turn tends to tip the tooth (Fig. 5). In this case the magnitude of the moment about the point CR will equal the force times the perpendicular distance from the centre of rotation to the line of action of the force. As another example, consider one implant supporting a single crown that is loaded vertically, but at a point C which is not on the centre line of the implant (Fig. 6). Here, in addition to an axial force, there will also be a moment on the implant equal to the

magnitude of the force times the perpendicular distance between the line of action of the force and the implant's centre. Although in formal mechanics a moment is a vector quantity, it serves our purposes now to simply speak of the moment about a point as being a scalar quantity equal to the force times the perpendicular distance between the point and the force's lines of action.

Survey of typical and maximum biting forces

Normal human patients with no oral implants or dentures can typically exert axial components of biting forces in the range of 100 to 2400 N (27 to 550 lbs) (Table I). The exact values depend on the patient, location in the mouth, nature of the food, chewing versus swallowing, degree of exertion, etc. Here, the term "axial" refers to the force component acting parallel to the long axis of a natural tooth (or implant), as discussed previously in relation to Fig. 1. Sometimes, the terms "vertical" or "occluso-apical" are used synonymously with "axial".

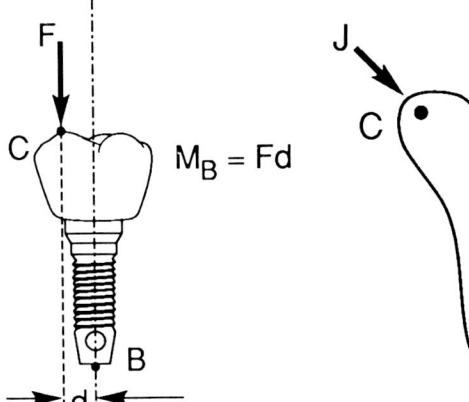

Fig. 6. Example of a moment being produced on an implant due to so-called eccentric loading: the point at which the force is applied (C) is at a distance d from the centre line of the implant.

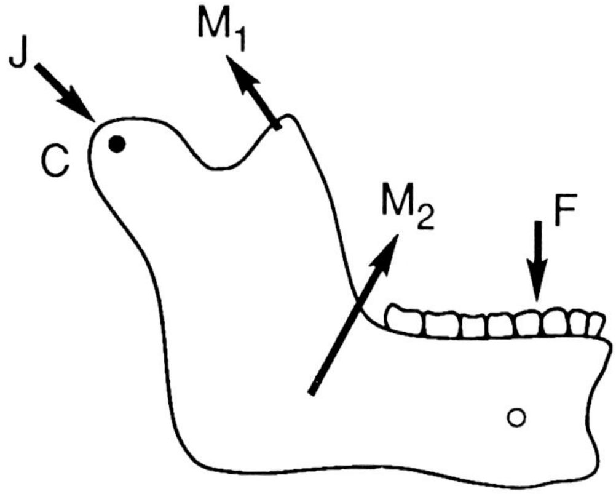

Fig. 7. Simplified model of the jaw as a class 3 lever. The fulcrum is at the condyle (C); while the two major muscle forces (M_1 and M_2) act nearer to the fulcrum than the biting force F. (J is the joint reaction force.)

Axial force components on natural teeth tend to be larger as one moves distally in the mouth. The explanation comes from a simple model of the mandible as a class 3 lever, in which all forces – i.e. those due to biting, the temporomandibular joint (TMJ) and jaw muscles – are assumed to act in the same plane, namely the sagittal plane. The lines of action of the forces due to the main muscles of mastication are distal to the point where the bite force typically occurs, and the fulcrum of the lever is at the TMJ (note point C in Fig. 7). This class 3 lever has a mechanical advantage of less than one, and the bite force will be larger if it acts nearer to the fulcrum, i.e. towards the TMJ. More sophisticated mathematical models of the jaw exist, but this class 3 lever model is sufficient as a starting point.

Typical magnitudes of axial forces are available from many sources (Table I). These data should be regarded as estimates for the typical magnitudes of axial forces on natural teeth in humans. The main limitation of these data is that the experimental techniques by which they were obtained involved the use of relatively large measuring devices such as bite forks or bite wafers. Such devices sometimes interfere with and change the details of chewing, so that the resulting data do not necessarily pertain to natural chewing events. Accordingly, much of the data in Table I represent what might best be termed as "closure forces", i.e. forces exerted on an object when the patient clamps the teeth on it. A closure force would tend to be axially directed, but its point of action and line of action can be uncertain in these types of measurements. This is because the bite force transducer is sometimes so large that more than one tooth is involved in the biting event; consequently, there are a few points (not just one) at which forces are acting. Nevertheless, the data in Table I at least provide reasonable estimates of expected biting forces *in vivo*.

Data on the lateral force components in the

natural or restored human dentition are scarce. One study reported that typical lateral components were about 20 N in the case of subjects with a prosthesis in the first mandibular molar region. This magnitude appears small compared to the typical axial force components in Table I. In view of the earlier discussion on resolving forces into axial and lateral components; and the influence of the curved surfaces of teeth (Fig. 1), it is reasonable to allow for the possibility that the lateral components could exceed 20 N. For instance, a bite force of 200 N acting at 45° to the long axis of an implant would have a lateral component equal to 141 N (= 200 N x cos 45°). Biting is clearly a dynamic (time-varying) process rather than a static event. Table I shows that the maximum closure speed of the mandible relative to the maxilla is estimated at about 140 mm/second. Nevertheless, most authorities believe that dynamics and related inertial effects do not appreciably affect biting loads, i.e. analyses based on statics are probably sufficient for most purposes. The net "chewing time per meal" has been found to be about 450 seconds. If the chewing frequency is about 1 Hz with a 0.3 second duration of tooth contact during each chewing stroke, there will be about 9 minutes per day during which chewing forces will act on teeth. If other activities such as swallowing are considered, the time might increase to about 17.5 minutes per day. Parafunctional habits such as bruxism would obviously increase this time. These estimates provide a useful indication of the minimum time per day that teeth (and perhaps implants) are load-bearing due to mastication and related events. For the restored dentition (Table I), completely edentulous patients who have soft tissue-supported dentures in both arches tend to bite with less axial force than patients with natural teeth or a denture oppos-

ing natural teeth. While individuals wearing complete maxillary and/or mandibular dentures have often shown an impaired ability to bite on solid objects, it may be possible for them to exert higher local loading levels than dentate patients if there is a balanced support of the denture.

For edentulous patients restored with full-arch prostheses supported by Brånemark implants, axial closure forces were found to be approximately equal to the forces in the normal dentate patient (Table I).

Predicting forces on oral implants

Statement of the problem

Assuming that the biting forces on a prosthesis are known, it is not always a simple matter to compute the loadings on the individual supporting abutments (natural teeth or implants). In general, these forces will not be the same as those exerted on the prosthesis. A simple example illustrates this point (Fig. 8). A downward force P acts at the end of a bridge with a cantilever section of length a. The distance between the line of action of P and the nearest implant (no. 2 in Fig. 8) is a. The bridge is assumed to be a rigid beam, supported by two implants (no. 1 and no. 2) spaced b apart. The problem is to predict the forces on implants no. 1 and no. 2.

A proper analysis begins with a so-called free body diagram of the beam (Fig. 8). The beam is isolated (removed from the implants) and all forces that act on the beam are shown. F_1 and F_2 represent the forces that the implants exert on the beam. (The directions of the forces, in the positive or in the negative direction of the y-axis in Fig. 8,

Table I. Bite forces and related data.

Description of the data	Typical values	Reference
(1) Vertical component of biting force in adults, averaged over several teeth	200–2440 N	Craig[4]
(2) Vertical component of biting force in adults, molar region	390–880 N	Craig[4]
(3) Vertical component of biting force in adults, premolar region	453 N	Craig[4]
(4) Vertical component of biting force in adults, incisor region	222 N	Craig[4]
(5) Vertical component of biting force in adults wearing complete dentures	77–196 N	Meng and Rugh[5], Ralph[6], Colaizzi et al.[7], Haraldson et al.[8]
(6) Vertical component of biting force in adults with a maxillary denture opposed by natural teeth in the mandible	147–284 N	Meng and Rugh[5]
(7) Vertical component of biting force in adults with dentures supported by implants (patients asked to exert max. force)	42–412 N (median 143 N)	Carlsson and Haraldson[9]
(8) Vertical component of biting force in adults with dentures supported by overdenture attachments	337–342 N	Meng and Rugh[5]
(9) Lateral components of biting forces in adults	~20 N	Graf[10]
(10) Frequency of chewing strokes	60–80 strokes/min	Harrison and Lewis[11]
(11) Rate of chewing	1–2 strokes/sec	Ahlgren,[12] Graf,[13]
(12) Duration of tooth contact in one chewing cycle	0.23–0.3 sec	Graf[13]
(13) Total time of tooth contact in a 24-hour period	9–17.5 min	Graf[13]
(14) Maximum closure speed of jaws during chewing	140 mm/sec	Harrison and Lewis[11]
(15) Maximum contact stresses on teeth	20 MPa	Carlsson[14]

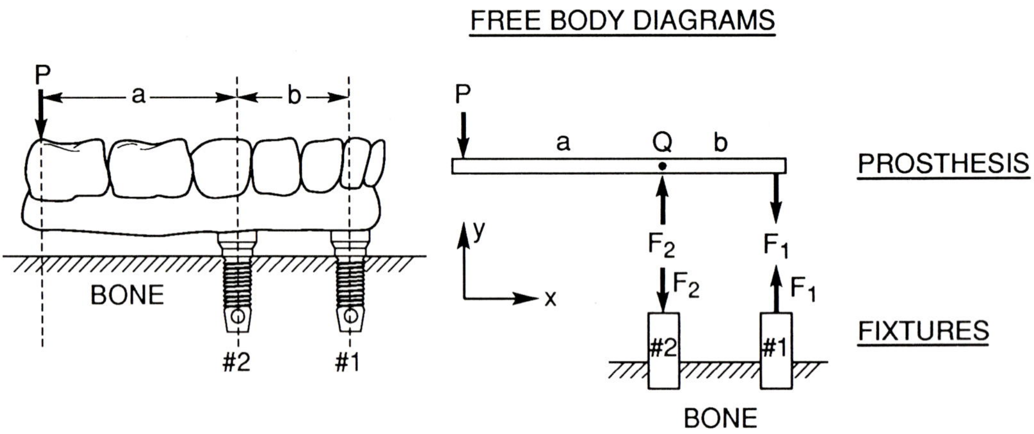

FREE BODY DIAGRAMS

Fig. 8. A method for predicting the forces on two implants supporting a cantilever portion of a prosthesis.

do not have to be known at this stage; the correct directions emerge from the solution.) Force P is the biting force. The second step is to recognize that the beam is in static equilibrium; according to Newton's laws this means that the sum of the forces and the sum of the moments on the beam are both zero. Finally, to solve for the two unknown forces F_1 and F_2, we write two equations which express the conditions of static equilibrium (note sign conventions according to the coordinate system in Fig. 8):

$$\Sigma F_y = 0: -F_1 + F_2 - P = 0.$$
$$\Sigma M_Q = 0: -F_1 b + aP = 0$$

The notation ΣF_y means summation of forces in the y-direction, while ΣM_Q means summation of moments about point Q. The solution of these two equations in two unknowns is $F_2 = (1+a/b)P$ and $F_1 = (a/b)P$. Therefore, although the bridge is loaded by the downward biting force P, the implants are loaded by forces whose magnitudes are larger than P, depending on the ratio a/b. That is, for a/b = 2, which is not uncommon in clinical practice, the forces on the implants are 3P and 2P. In understanding the

direction in which these forces act, note the difference in the directions of F_1 and F_2 according to whether one looks at the free body diagram of the bridge or the free body diagram of the implants (Fig. 8). The forces on the bridge from the implants are equal but opposite to the forces on the implants from the bridge (Newton's third law: for every action there is an equal and opposite reaction). In any case, the forces F_1 and F_2 do not act in the same direction. Implant no. 2, nearest to the point at which P acts, experiences a compressive load, tending to push it into the bone. Implant no. 1 experiences a tensile load, tending to pull it out of the bone.

The general problem of calculating the forces on more than two implant abutments supporting a loaded prosthesis is more involved. There may be many complicating factors, including:

(1) The nature of mastication, e.g. frequency of chewing, strength of biting, sequence of the chewing cycle, favoured-side biting, mandibular movements;

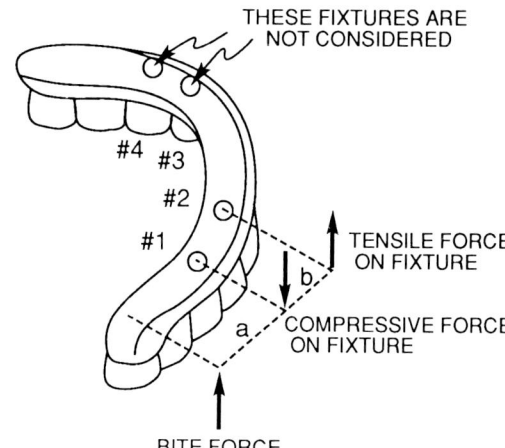

THESE FIXTURES ARE
NOT CONSIDERED

#4 #3

#2

#1

TENSILE FORCE
ON FIXTURE

b

a

COMPRESSIVE FORCE
ON FIXTURE

BITE FORCE

Fig. 9. Diagrammatic view of a maxillary prosthesis loaded by a biting force. Forces at implant locations no. 1 and no. 2 can be predicted approximately by the method used in Fig. 8, provided implants at locations no. 3 and no. 4 are assumed not to participate.

(2) The nature of the prosthesis, e.g. full or partial dentures, tissue-supported versus implant-supported prostheses, number and location of implants and teeth, angulation of implants;

(3) The biomechanical properties of the structures and materials comprising the bridge or prosthesis, implants and bone, e.g. elastic moduli, structural stiffnesses, nature of the connection between implant and bridge (cemented versus screwed), and deformability of the mandible or maxilla.

Methods to account for some of these factors are discussed below. Note that all calculation methods are based on some type of idealization, or model, of reality. Consequently, the clinician must understand the underlying assumptions of a particular model and consider its limitations with respect to a given clinical situation.

Models for predicting loads on implants

The simplest model of a dental prosthesis is to regard it as a straight, rigid beam, as discussed by *Rangert* et al.[15]. In fact, their model was already illustrated in the example above, with a cantilever-type bridge supported by two implants (Fig. 8). For a more realistic case of, say, four maxillary implants supporting a maxillary framework in the Brånemark system (Fig. 9), the Rangert model only considers the pair of implants closest to the applied bite force. The distances a and b could be measured at the chairside. Then, the forces on the two implants nearest to the applied force P can be obtained as in the previous example (Fig. 8). However, the limitation of this model is that it does not predict forces on all four implants; the model predicts that the two implants nearest the applied load P are "doing all the work". Clearly; this is just an assumption of the model; it may not be true. While this seems to be a serious limitation of this model, there is evidence that the model is an acceptable approximation to

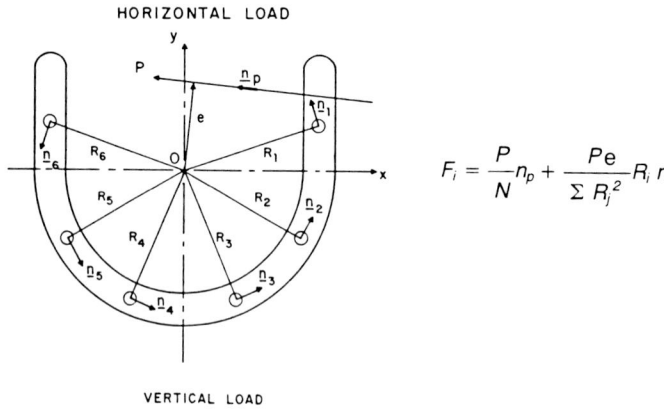

$$F_i = \frac{P}{N} n_p + \frac{Pe}{\Sigma R_j^2} R_i\, n_i$$

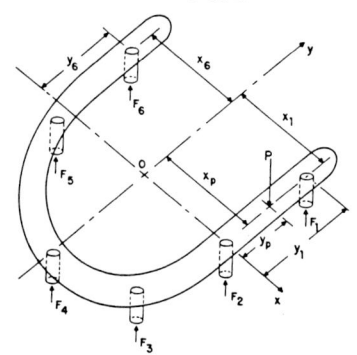

$$F_i = \frac{P}{N} + P(Ax_i + By_i)$$

Fig. 10. The Skalak model: given the number and arrangement of implants and the bridge load P, the horizontal and vertical forces on each fixture are computed using the equations shown. (A more complete discussion of the equations appears in references [3] and [16].)

reality when there is a certain amount of deformability in the framework and in the connections between framework and abutments. As a rule, in a multi-implant situation, the *Rangert* model will tend to overestimate the loads on the two implants nearest to the applied load P.

The problem of predicting loads on *all* of the abutments in a multi-implant distribution is a statically indeterminate problem in mechanics. This means that the abutment loadings cannot be obtained using only the theory of rigid body statics (i.e. the underlying theory of the *Rangert* model). However, it is possible to solve a statically indeterminate problem if information about the mechanical properties of the bridge, abutments, and interfacial tissues is avail-

able. The model developed by *Skalak*[16] was the first solution of this sort for dental prostheses.

Skalak's model is based on an established method used to predict the load distribution among bolts or rivets holding plates together. When applied to the oral implant situation, the model can predict the vertical and horizontal force components on implants supporting a bridge subjected to vertical and horizontal loadings (Fig. 10). It is assumed that the bridge and bone are rigid, but that the implants and/or their connections to bridge and/or bone are elastic. *Skalak*'s model predicts that a purely verti cal force on the prosthesis (i.e. acting perpendicular to the plane of the prosthesis) is counterbalanced by a distribution of purely vertical forces among the N supporting abutments. Similarly, for a horizontal load on the prosthesis (i.e. acting in the plane of the prosthesis), the model predicts that there will be a counterbalancing distribution of horizontal forces among the N abutments. The equations for calculating these forces are summarized in Fig. 10. Generally, an arbitrary force vector on the prosthesis will have both vertical and horizontal components. In this case, the model predicts that there will be both vertical and horizontal force components on each of the implants. The detailed equations from the model are used to make separate calculations of the implant loadings due to the vertical and horizontal loading components of the applied force on the prosthesis. The total loading on each implant is the combined result of the vertical and horizontal load components.

Some sample results computed by the *Skalak* model provide useful illustrations. Consider two cases: four or six implants symmetrically distributed about the midline of a mandible over the same arc of 112.5°, with the radius of the mandible equal to 22.5 mm. The arc of 112.5° represents a distance roughly equal to that between the mental foramina in the human mandible. The problem is to predict the vertical forces on each implant when a single vertical force of magnitude 30 N acts at a position defined by $\theta = 10°$ (Fig. 11).

First, for the six-implant case with a vertical load of 30 N at $\theta = 10°$ (a case of cantilever loading), the most distal implants nearest the load (no. 1, 2) experience compressive forces (negative values) as does implant no. 6, on the other side of the prosthesis. Meanwhile, the three anterior implants (no. 3, 4 and 5) experience tensile forces (positive values). This result can be understood by recognizing that the implants are exerting forces on the bridge to keep it from

tipping distally and to the side under the action of the applied cantilever loading. Note that for the applied vertical load magnitude of 30 N, the loads on the implants are less than 30 N, except for that on implant no. 1 nearest the loading point, which is about −40 N (the negative sign indicates compression). Since this model is linear, we can obtain the results for a different applied vertical load – say 100 N – by multiplying the above data by 100/30.

Now, to compare the six-implant case above with a four-implant case, consider the results for four implants distributed over the same arc as the six implants (112.5°). The results (Fig. 11) show that the magnitudes of the forces on the most distal implants are similar in both cases. This means that there is only a slight difference between using four implants and six implants to support a prosthesis, when the four implants are spaced out over the same arc as the six implants. Note that the inter-implant spacing in the four-implant case is larger than in the six-implant case; this compensates for fewer implants, which would otherwise tend to increase the loading per implant. To make this point more clearly, consider now a new arrangement of four implants, created by removing the two most distal implants from the six-implant case above, keeping the inter-implant spacing the same. In this instance, the forces on the four remaining implants become much larger than in the original six-implant case (Fig. 12). It can be shown that an even worse situation is four implants positioned in a straight line across the anterior of the mandible; this results in even larger forces per implant when the prosthesis is loaded by a vertical force in the distal region. In terms of the more approximate model of *Rangert* et al., this case illustrates a situation with a very large ratio a/b owing to the fact that b is very small.

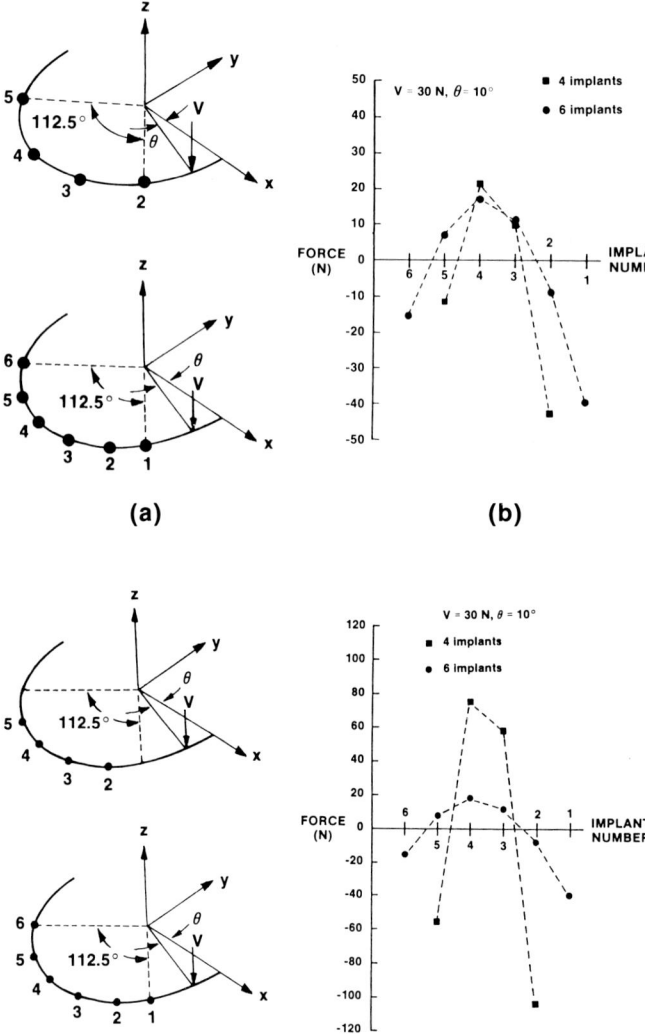

Fig. 11. Results from the *Skalak* model. The four-implant case (top) has a larger inter-implant spacing than the six-implant case. The plots in (b) show that the magnitude of the forces on the implants is about equal in the six- and four-implant cases.

Fig. 12. Results from the *Skalak* model. Implants no. 1 and no. 6 have been removed from the six-implant arrangement in (a), yielding a four-implant arrangement with the same inter-implant spacing as the original six-implant case. The plots in (b) show that the forces are higher in the four-implant case.

An important point is that the models above do not specifically consider the effects of implant angulation. For example, consider the original simple model of a bridge with a cantilever, but with the modification that implant no. 1 is inclined to the vertical by 30° (Fig. 13). The solution to the problem is unchanged; the only difference is that the force on implant no. 1 causes an off-axis loading of the implant. (The reader should recall the concept of resolving a force into components.) Although, clearly, this situation could lead to problems with either the implant or the bone (or perhaps both), the nature of these problems is a separate discussion, not directly addressed by either the *Skalak* or the *Rangert* models. Nevertheless, these models are a starting point. More recent analysis of forces on implants supporting bridgework have been accom-

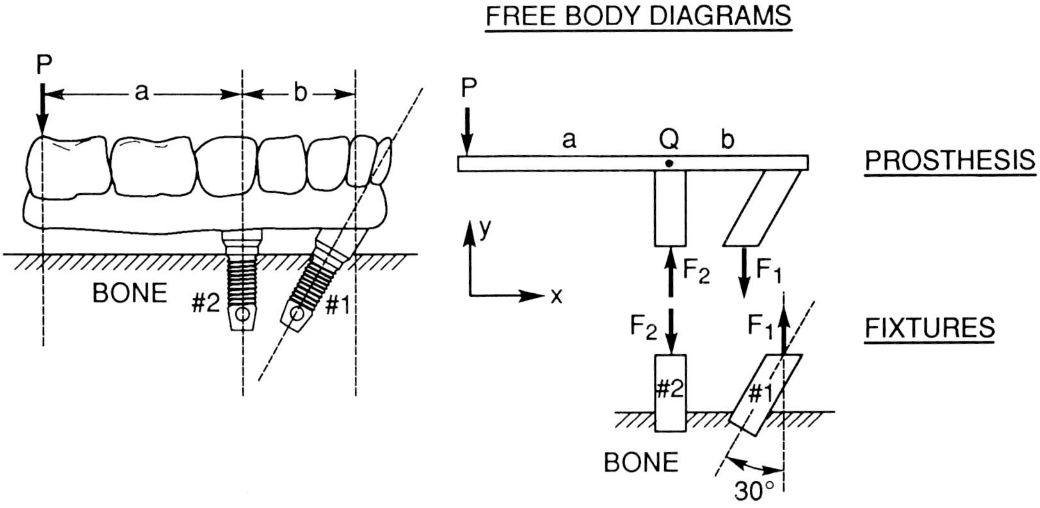

FREE BODY DIAGRAMS

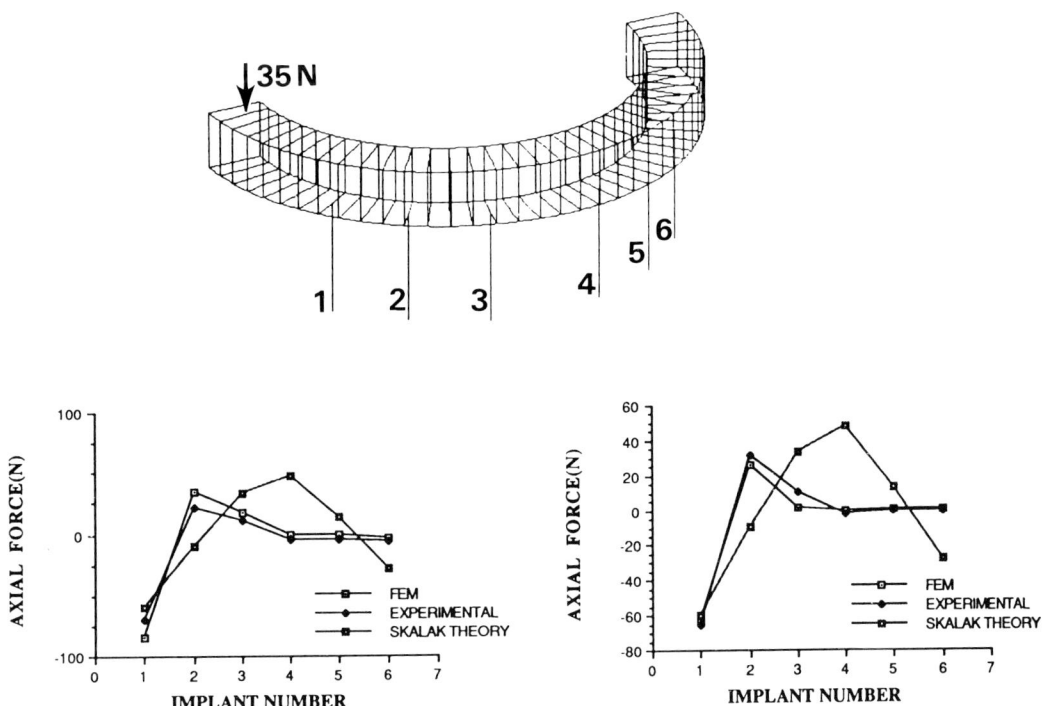

Fig. 13. Same diagram as for Fig. 7, except that one of the implants here has a 30° inclination. There will be a significant lateral force component on implant. No. 1.

Fig. 14 A finite element model (top) used to predict forces on six implants supporting a full-arch prosthesis. Plots on the left and right show axial forces on the implants when the prosthesis is metal or acrylic, respectively[17].

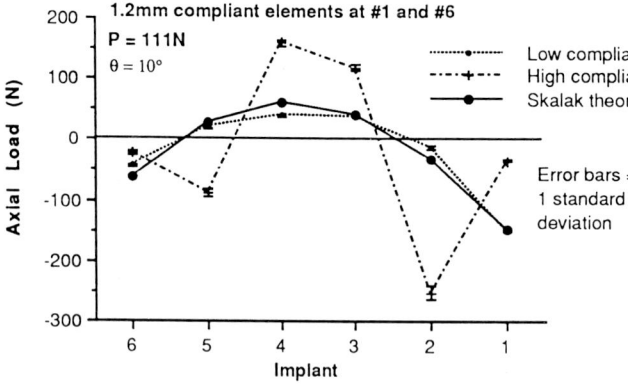

Fig. 15. This shows the changes in the force distribution among abutments, relative to predictions of the Skalak model, when implants no. 1 and no. 6 have about 10x lower stiffness (i.e. are more compliant) than implants no. 2, 3, 4, and 5. The effect is to increase the forces on implants no. 2, 3, 4 and 5.

plished by a powerful computer method called finite element modeling (FEM). FE models can account for properties of the prosthesis, position and angulation of implants, properties of the interfacial bone, etc. For example, a recent model[17] showed that the structural rigidity of the prosthesis (which depends on the elastic modulus, the shape and the dimensions of the prosthesis), as well as the stiffness of the bone–implant connections, can affect force distribution among the implants. For instance, in a cantilever loading case, the load distribution did not exactly follow the predictions of the *Skalak* model for an acrylic prosthesis or for a metallic prosthesis (Fig. 14). The *Skalak* model assumes that the prosthesis is infinitely rigid, which is obviously not quite accurate for the two prostheses examined in Fig. 14. Evidently, the acrylic and metal alloy bridge show a degree of flexibility, which has the effect of concentrating forces on those implants nearest to the loading point. FE models also show that things become more complicated when all of the abutments do not have the same stiffnesses (spring constants). When

this is the case, it becomes difficult to generalize about the results, except to say that the stiffest implants in the distribution will generally take most of the load, all other things being equal. For example, in cantilever loading, a six-implant distribution will start to behave more like a four-implant distribution if two of the six original implants become less stiff (Fig. 15). (The decrease in stiffness might be caused by weakening of interfacial bone or formation of interfacial fibrous tissue.)

The above discussion leads naturally to a more in-depth consideration of tooth and implant stiffness and biomechanical analyses related to the use of implants in partially edentulous patients.

Stiffness of teeth and implants

The stiffness of a tooth or implant is related to the clinical term mobility. Mobility as discussed here does not mean orthodontically-induced tooth movements, resulting from biological activities around a tooth or implant. Instead it means relatively small

COMPARATIVE AXIAL "STIFFNESS"

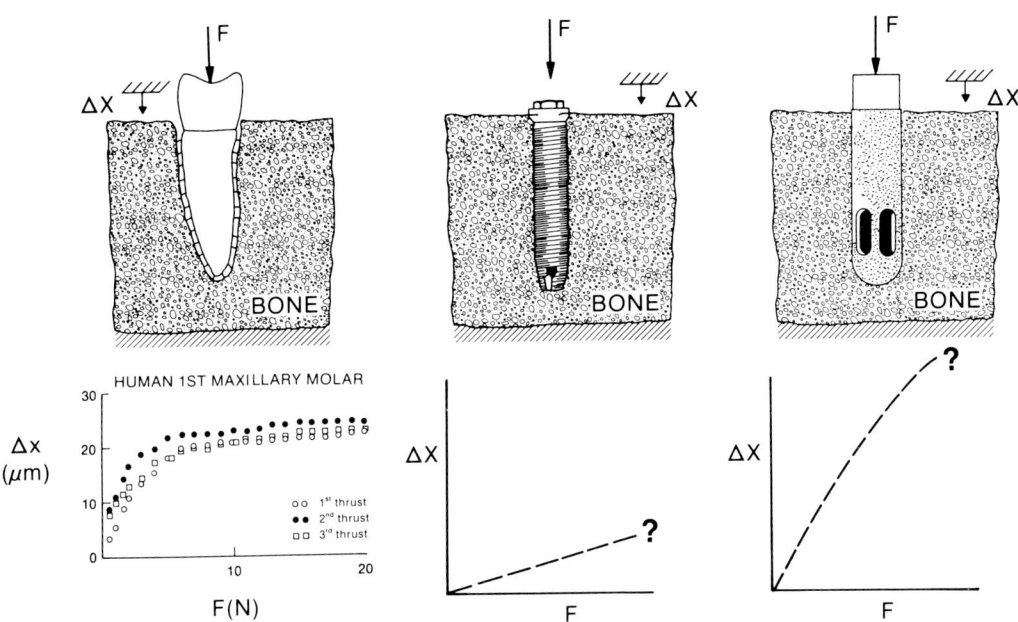

Fig. 16. Characteristics of tooth[24] and implant mobility in the axial direction.

(e.g. tenths or thousandths of a mm), reversible displacements of teeth or implants caused by applied forces. Clinically, mobility describes how a tooth or implant moves with respect to a fixed reference under the action of an applied force. When testing tooth mobility, a dentist typically applies a lateral force to a tooth with a dental instrument (say a mirror handle) and then estimates the movement of the tooth by eye. Movement greater than, say, 1 mm is easily detected and would suggest an advanced degree of breakdown in the periodontal support system of the tooth.

Now, if one considers a prosthesis supported by both teeth and implants, the difficulty is that teeth and implants do not have the same mobility characteristics and, in any case, neither the Rangert nor Skalak models explicitly deal with differing mobilities among abutments. (However, a new version of the original Skalak model is being developed by the authors to consider different mobilities among the abutments). Nevertheless, a review of the literature on tooth and implant mobility leads to a definition of stiffness and a way to approach this problem.

First, teeth and implants can be displaced in different directions: intrusively, extrusively, laterally, mesiodistally, or combinations thereof. Sometimes there may be tooth displacements in more than one direction, even when the applied force only acts in one direction, but this can be ignored as a secondary effect. Secondly, when a constant force is applied to a tooth or implant, the displacement of the tooth or implant may increase slowly with time; this phenomenon is called creep. With implants, creep is probably not significant unless there is fibrous tissue around the implant (Table II).[19] Thirdly, intrusive tooth displacement is not always linear with intrusive force

Table II. Data on intrusive stiffnesses of dental implants and teeth, *in vitro* and *in vivo*

Test conditions	Stiffness (N/µm)	References
(1) *Implant alone, no interfacial tissue*		
• IMZ implant with IME, TIE and gold screw	2.57	*Hoshaw* and *Brunski*[18]
• Flexiroot with polymer insert and attachment	4.11	"
• Brånemark fixture (7 mm) plus abutment screw, abutment and gold cylinder	4.55	"
• Driskell Bioengineering (Stryker) implant, with abutment	5.50	"
(2) *Implants in tissues or tissue analogs, in vitro*		
• Brånemark (7 mm) in trabecular bone (bovine tibial metaphysis)	2.50	"
• Brånemark in polycarbonate plastic	3.66	"
• Ti Blade-Vent implant in fibrous tissue, dog mandible	0.22–0.88	*Brunski* and *Schock*[19]
• Bioglass cylindrical implants in fibrous tissue, dog mandible	1.9	*Weinstein* et al.[20]
• Bioglass cylindrical implants with a direct bone–implant interface, dog mandible	8.5	"
(3) *Implants, in vivo*		
• Tübingen Al_2O_3 implant, human mandible	10	*Schulte*[21]
(4) *Natural teeth, in vivo*		
• Human molar	0.1–1.0	*Richter* et al.[22]
• Human incisor	0.1–3.0	*Picton*[23]
• "Tooth 24"	0.1–1.0	*Schulte*[21]

(Fig. 16). Data for a maxillary incisor show that there is an approximately bilinear relationship between intrusive displacement and intrusive force on a tooth. The tooth displaces less per unit load when loaded beyond about 49 N.

In arriving at a definition of stiffness, it is first necessary to define displacement. Displacement is a vector quantity, having both magnitude and direction. For example, if one pushes laterally with a 1 N force on the tip of a tooth, the tip might move (displace) 0.2 mm in a direction parallel to the applied force. Alternatively, one might apply the 1 N force in a different direction – e.g. parallel to the tooth's long axis, an intrusive force – causing an intrusive displacement measuring 0.1 mm. In either case, a coordinate system is needed to describe both the force and the displacement. Typically, one picks an x-y-z coordinate system that is fixed with respect to some reference point such as a nearby section of jaw bone.

Although the data given above on tooth and

implant mobility show that they do not behave exactly like simple springs, for many purposes this idealization (or model) is sufficient as an approximation. That is; when a force **F** is applied to a tooth or implant, the displacement from its equilibrium position Δx is related to the force by the following simple equation:

$$F = k\Delta x \qquad (6)$$

in which k is a spring constant, or stiffness. The stiffness k depends on the material and structural properties of the tooth or implant and the mechanical properties of the tissues in which the tooth or implant resides. Assuming that the tooth or implant stiffness is one spring (with spring constant k_{tooth} or $k_{implant}$) attached in series with a second spring; representing the tissue interface (with spring constant $k_{interface}$), then these two springs in series have the net spring constant, k_{net}, given by:

$$1/k_{net} = 1/k_{implant} + 1/k_{interface} \qquad (7)$$

Table II shows typical stiffness data for teeth and implants taken from a variety of sources. Values of about 3–5 N/μm have been determined for the net spring stiffness of an IMZ system including an intra-mobile element (IME). Most implants in bone produce a net stiffness greater than for natural teeth; in Table II the largest value of 10 N/μm is for an alumina implant in bone. However, if there is a soft tissue interface around an implant (Table II)[19, 20], then the stiffness values are similar to those of natural teeth; but less than those for implants with an osseointegrated interface.

Models for predicting forces on prostheses supported by teeth and implants

Based on the stiffness concept, the distribution of forces among natural teeth and implants supporting a prosthesis can now be considered again.

Illustrative analyses can be done by finite element methods[25] for the case of a prosthesis supported by a natural tooth and one implant with or without an "intra-mobile element". The natural teeth and implants can be represented in the FE model as having the same size and shape but different mechanical properties and support. Teeth were modelled as dentin surrounded by a periodontal ligament. The bone around implants and teeth was assumed to be homogeneous and isotropic. The stiffness of a natural tooth in the FE model was 1.17 N/μm, which approximates to the mid-range stiffness value of a natural tooth (Table II). For implants made of titanium but with no IME, the stiffness was 12.5 N/μm, which is within the high range for implant–bone stiffness (Table II). For implants with a built-in IME, the stiffness was 8.33 N/μm. This decrease in stiffness from 12.5 to 8.33 N/μm showed at the outset that an implant will indeed become less stiff when an IME is incorporated, in agreement with the design rationale for an IMZ-type implant. However, the question is whether this makes much of a difference (see below).

The results of the FE analysis of the prosthesis supported by two abutments illustrates typical findings (Fig. 17). The prosthesis was loaded in the middle by a single vertical force of 100 N. The results showed that the natural tooth supported about 30% of the total vertical force when it was paired with a pure titanium implant with no IME. However, when an IME was incorporated within the implant, the tooth sup-

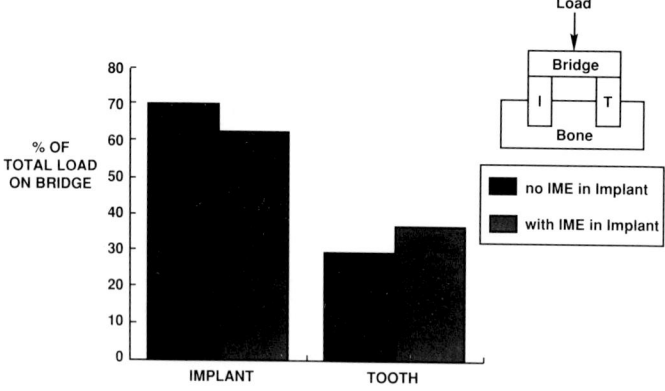

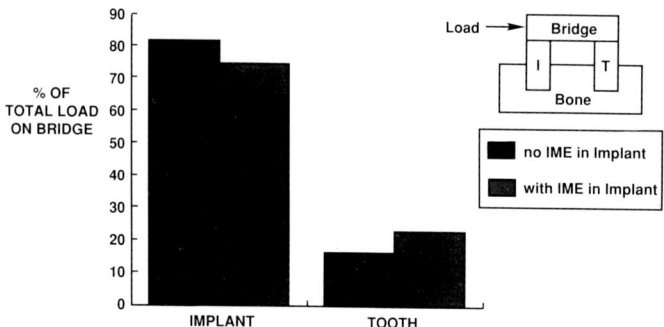

Fig. 17. Finite element results showing changes in the load sharing (axial and lateral) between a tooth and implant when the implant does, or does not, have a built-in intra-mobile element.

ported a slightly larger share, i.e. about 38%, of the force applied to the prosthesis. For a total horizontal force of 25 N applied to the bridge at either the mesial or distal end, 18% of the total load was taken by the tooth when the implant was pure titanium, but this decreased to 25% when the implant contained an IME.

These results are consistent with the rationale for the use of an IME in an implant; since the IME decreased the force on the implant and increased the force on the tooth, as compared to the case of an implant with no IME. However, since the changes were small, it is not evident from this model whether this would have much effect in the clinical situation.

Rangert et al.[26] also analysed the problem of a prosthesis supported by a natural tooth and one osseointegrated implant. They presented data indicating a small but significant degree of flexibility in the entire mechanical system, which consisted of the prosthesis and the abutment screw joint of the Brånemark system. Then, using this data and related calculations, they estimated the load-sharing between a tooth and an implant. Overall, they reached the same conclusion as noted in the FE study above, namely that there was a relatively equal sharing of force between the tooth and the implant, even when there was no IME in the implant. Therefore, the need for an IME inside an osseointegrated implant is questionable from a biomechanical point of view.

As mentioned earlier, in the case of a prosthesis supported by several abutments; each with different stiffnesses, the force distribution among the abutments is difficult to predict. Experiments in the laboratory show, for example, that if low-stiffness abutments are located bilaterally at the two most distal locations in a six-implant distribution, they support essentially none of the applied load, while the other four; higher-stiffness implants support most of the load. In effect, the six-implant distribution becomes more like a four-implant distribution (Fig. 15).

Biomechanics of frameworks and misfit

Frameworks

The metal framework used in a typical full-arch prosthesis with the Brånemark system can sometimes fracture *in vivo*. Unfortunately, no in depth analyses of such fractures, including case histories and explanations, exist. Nevertheless, it is possible to suggest some reasons for these fractures, based on the biomechanical analyses presented so far. Fractures have been observed to occur more towards the cantilever sections of the framework, for example, just distal to the most distal implant. The fractures could be caused by two mechanisms. One is outright overload of the cantilever by a single vertical bite force; the

distal portion of the prosthesis may bend like a cantilever beam and eventually fracture at the root of the cantilever, where the stress is greatest. However, this mode of fracture is unlikely in a reasonably-sized prosthesis made of a typical prosthetic alloy. The force needed to induce fracture-level stresses in the beam would be much larger than the typical biting forces of a few hundred newtons. A more likely reason for prosthesis fracture is metallurgical fatigue under cyclic biting loads. The stresses in the prosthesis caused by the cyclic forces of chewing day after day could produce stresses at the root of the cantilever which exceed the fatigue limit of the prosthetic alloy. To forestall such failures, the cross-sectional area of the framework near the root of the cantilever should be relatively substantial, i.e. in the order of 3–6 mm on a side. This will help to reduce bending stresses in this region because the stress varies with the square of the thickness of the beam and linearly with its width.

Gold screws and abutment screws

Other types of failure may involve the screw joints in for example the Brånemark system. The metal framework of a full-arch prosthesis is held onto the abutments by screw joints, in which the gold screw is torqued into the abutment screw. The screw joint's main function is to clamp the gold cylinder and attached framework onto the abutment cylinder[26]. The biomechanics of the screw joint are important in determining the loading of the component parts and the propensity for failure in various parts of the system.

Ideally, when the gold screw is torqued into the abutment screw at the prescribed torque, the torque T (nominally 10 N·cm) causes a tensile force in the gold screw and abutment screw and a compressive clamping force on the titanium abutment cylinder. The two forces are equal and opposite and hold the joint closed; this is the desired situation in the screw joint. According to machine theory, there is a relationship between the applied torque T and the tensile force **F** in the screw, according to the equation:

$$T = \kappa DF \qquad (8)$$

Here, κ is a dimensionless constant whose value depends on such factors as screw thread geometry and friction at interfaces; D is the screw diameter. Under ideal conditions, in for example the Brånemark system, the applied torque of 10 N·cm on the gold screw produces a tensile force of about 300 N in the flat-headed gold screw (and in the titanium abutment screw to which it is attached) and an equal compressive force on the gold cylinder and titanium abutment[26, 27]. (The force is 160 N when the old-style conical-head gold screw is used.) This joint-clamping force is called the preload.

The significance of the preload is that the screw joint will start to open if the externally applied force on the gold cylinder exceeds approximately 300 N in tension. However, the value of 300 N pertains to ideal conditions in the screw joint, and non-ideal conditions can occur clinically. Examples of non-ideal conditions include uneven, pitted or damaged mating surfaces of the gold screw and gold cylinder. Under such non-ideal conditions, the preload may decrease to less than 200 N, even though the nominal torque of 10 N·cm is applied during tightening of the joint.[27] In effect, the surface imperfections increase the value of κ in Eq. (8); as κ is increased, the preload (**F**) will be less for the same tightening torque (T). This

is significant because it means that a non-ideal joint will begin to open at forces less than the ideal value of 300 N, i.e. at 150 to 200 N. Since it is quite possible for tensile forces of 150 N to occur on implants in anterior locations when a prosthesis has significant cantilevers, it is possible that joint opening may be more of a clinical problem than has hitherto been realized.

Framework misfit

Most frameworks for full-arch prostheses are made using impressions, plaster models, and casting techniques, etc. Despite every effort at precision, dimensional inaccuracies inevitably occur in the final cast metal framework. Assuming that the misfit is not too severe, the framework may appear (at least by visual inspection) to fit well "passively", onto the abutments. However, there is increasing concern about the assessment of "passive fit" and its clinical significance.

A working definition of passive fit is suggested by a free body diagram (Fig. 18). This shows a framework for five abutments. Suppose four of the five abutments match perfectly with the gold cylinders in the framework. Assume that when each of the gold screws is torqued down onto the well-fitting abutments, the ideal preload of 300 N develops in each joint. However, suppose one of the five abutments does not fit well; note the gap (exaggerated, to make the point) between one of the abutments and the framework in Fig. 18. Now, as the gold screw is torqued down to 10 N·cm at the site of the gap, the tension which develops in the gold screw and abutment screw will act on the framework, tending to bend it down toward the abutment, diminishing the gap. If the gap is small, it might be possible to close it completely by such deformation of

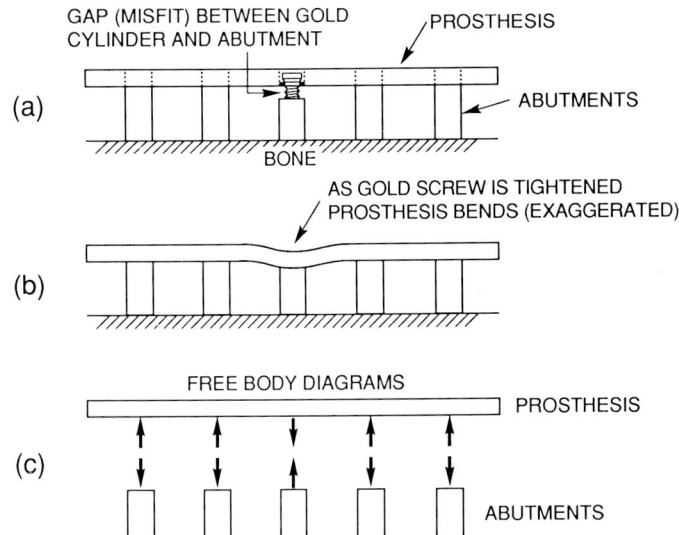

(a)

(b)

(c)

Fig. 18. Diagrammatic demonstration of how a misfitting framework can cause loads on implants even before any biting force is applied to the prosthesis.

the framework. However, if the gap is large, it may not be closed even when the nominal torque of 10 N·cm is reached. In either case, the net effect is to apply a force on the framework at the location of the misfit. This force can be considered as an "external" force acting on the framework as per the *Skalak* model; this means that the other four implants will be loaded by virtue of the force on the framework at the site of misfit. Although this is a reasonable theoretical explanation, clinical data on this effect are lacking.

Summary

Although the design of osseointegrated implants and prostheses is not yet an exact science, many biomechanical aspects can now be discussed quantitatively. Maximum biting forces on fixed prostheses are of the same order of magnitude as the vertical forces in the natural dentition, i.e. 100–1000 N, maximum. The distribution of loads applied by a prosthesis to the underlying implants is not precisely known, but predictions are available from approximate models. Without cantilevers, the maximum vertical force on any implant will generally be less than the bite force. With cantilevers, however, the maximum load on the implant nearest to the cantilever region may be two to three times the applied bite force, while the next implant may be under tension equal to one or perhaps two times the bite force. The flexibility of most implants and bridges is sufficient to allow direct connection of a bridge to both implants and natural teeth. Frameworks should be accurately made to ensure that the screw joints can be tightened to produce the maximum clamping force of about 300 N between the gold cylinders and the abutments. Ill-fitting frameworks should be avoided, because they can cause a load distribution on the implants, even before any biting forces act on the prosthesis.

References

[1] *Brånemark, P.-I., Zarb, G., Albrektsson, T.* (eds). Tissue integrated prostheses. Chicago: Quintessence Publ. Co., 1985.

[2] *Brunski, J. B.* Influence of biomechanical factors at the bone–biomaterial interface. In: *Davies, J. E.* (ed.) The bone–biomaterial interface. pp. 391–405. Toronto: University of Toronto Press, 1991.

[3] *Brunski, J. B.* Biomechanical factors affecting the bone–dental implant interface. Clin Mater 1992; *10:* 153–201.

[4] *Craig, R. G.* (ed.). Restorative dental materials (6th edn). pp. 60–61. St. Louis, MO: C. V. Mosby, 1980.

[5] *Meng, T. R., Rugh, J. D.* Biting force on overdenture and conventional denture patients. J Dent Res 1983; *62:* 249 (Abstract No. 716).

[6] *Ralph, W. J.* The effects of dental treatment on biting force. J Prosth Dent 1979; *41:* 143.

[7] *Colaizzi, F. A., Javid, N. S., Michael, C. G., Gibbs, C. J.* Biting force, EMG, and jaw movements in denture wearers. J Dent Res 1984; *63:* 329 (Abstract No. 1424).

[8] *Haraldsson, T., Karlsson, U., Carlsson, G. E.* Bite force and oral function in complete denture wearers. J Oral Rehabil 1979; *6:* 41–48.

[9] *Carlsson, G. E., Haraldsson, T.* Functional response. In: *Brånemark, P.-I., Zarb, G., Albrektsson, T.* (eds). Tissue integrated prostheses. pp. 155–163. Chicago: Quintessence Publ. Co., 1985.

[10] *Graf, H.* Occlusal forces during function: In: *Rowe, N. H.* Occlusion: research on form and function. pp. 90–111. Ann Arbor: University of Michigan, 1975.

[11] *Harrison, A., Lewis, T. T.* The development of an abrasion testing machine. J Biomed Mater Res 1975, *9:* 341–353.

[12] *Ahlgren, J.* Mechanism of mastication. Acta Odontol Scand, 1966; *24,* (Suppl. 44): 100–104.

[13] *Graf, H.* Bruxism 1969; *16:* 659–665.

[14] *Carlsson, G. E.* Bite force and chewing efficiency. Front Oral Physiol 1974; *1:* 265–292.

[15] *Rangert, B., Jemt, T., Joneus, L.* Forces and moments on Brånemark implants. Int J Oral Maxillofac Implants 1989; *4:* 241–247.

[16] *Skalak, R.* Aspects of biomechanical considerations. In: *Brånemark, P.-I., Zarb, G., Albrektsson, T.* (eds). Tissue integrated prostheses. pp. 117–128. Chicago: Quintessence Publ. Co., 1985.

[17] *Elias, J. J., Brunski, J. B.* Finite element analysis of load distribution among dental implants. In: *Vanderby, R. Jr.* (ed.). pp. 155–158. 1991 Advances in bioengineering. BED Vol. 20, American Society of Mechanical Engineers, 1991.

[18] *Hoshaw, S. J., Brunski, J. B.* Mechanical testing of dental implants with and without "intramobile elements". J Dent Res 1988; *67:* 314 (abstract No. 1612).

[19] *Brunski, J. B., Schock, R. B.* Mechanical behavior of a fibrous tissue interface of an endosseous dental implant. Trans 5th Ann Meeting Soc for Biomaterials. p. 41.

[20] *Weinstein, A. M., Klawitter, J. J., Cook, S. D.* Implant–bone characteristics of bioglass dental implants. J Biomed Mater Res 1980; *14:* 23–29.

[21] *Schulte, W.* The intraosseous Al_2O_3 (Frialit) Tübingen implant). Developmental status after eight years (I). Quintessence Int 1984; *15:* 1–39.

[22] *Richter, E.-J., Orschall, B., Jovanovich, S. A.* Dental implant abutment resembling the two-phase tooth mobility. J Biomech 1990; *23:* 297–306.

[23] *Picton, D. C. A.* Vertical movement of teeth during biting. Arch Oral Biol 1963; *8:* 109–118.

[24] *Moxham, B. J., Berkovitz, B. K. B.* The effects of external forces on the periodontal ligament – the response to axial loads. In: *Berkovitz, B. K. B., Moxham, B. J., Newman, H. N.* (eds). The periodontal ligament in health and disease. pp. 249–268. Oxford: Pergamon Press, 1982.

[25] *El Wakad, M.* Measurement and prediction of loading on dental implants: transducer design and finite element modelling (Thesis). Department of Biomedical Engineering, Rensselaer Polytechnic Institute. Troy, NY, 1988.

[26] *Rangert, B., Gunne, J., Sullivan, D. Y.* Mechanical aspects of a Brånemark implant connected to a natural tooth: an *in vitro* study. Int J Oral Maxillofac Implants 1991; *6:* 177–186.

[27] *Carr, A. B., Brunski, J. B., Labishak, J., Bagley, B.* Preload comparison between as-received and cast-to implant cylinders. J Dent Res 1993; *72:* 190 (abstract No. 695).

Chapter 8

Fundamental principles of bone physiology, metabolism and loading

W. E. Roberts

As a result of unique physiological mechanisms, bone serves two antagonistic functions: structural support and calcium metabolism[8]. The strength of a bone (quantity, quality and distribution of osseous tissue) is directly related to loading[1]. As an energy conservation measure, bone that is not adequately loaded is resorbed, and the skeletal system continuously adapts to achieve optimal strength with minimal mass. The delicate structural balance is further challenged by metabolic function. An adequate reserve of osseous tissue must be maintained to provide a continuous stream of ionic calcium without compromising structural integrity. To provide for a variety of conflicting demands, the skeleton has evolved structural and metabolic fractions (Fig. 1).

Osteopenia (inadequate bone mass) is a common clinical problem. It may be due to functional atrophy and/or negative calcium balance. Prospective oral implant patients are likely to present with localized and systemic skeletal problems for three reasons:

(1) Bone in edentulous areas is usually atrophic;
(2) Metabolic bone disease is prevalent in middle-aged and older adults;[8]

(3) Integrated implants are often indicated for patients with a history of severe bone loss[12].

Modelling and remodelling

Unique mechanisms of bone adaptation have evolved to maintain structural integrity, repair fatigue damage, and provide a continuous source of metabolic calcium (Fig. 2). Modelling involves individual (uncoupled) sites of bone formation or resorption that change the shape or form of a bone. This is the principal mechanism for adapting osseous structure to functional loading. Remodelling is the mechanism of bone turnover. It involves coupled sequences of cell activation (A), bone resorption (R) and bone formation (F). The duration of the ARF remodelling cycle (sigma) is about 4 months in man[2].

Modelling is the principal means of skeletal adaptation to functional and therapeutic loads. Relatively modest changes in the distribution of osseous tissue along cortical bone surfaces can dramatically change the overall load-bearing capability. For instance, the stiffness of a long bone, such as the body of the mandible, is related to the

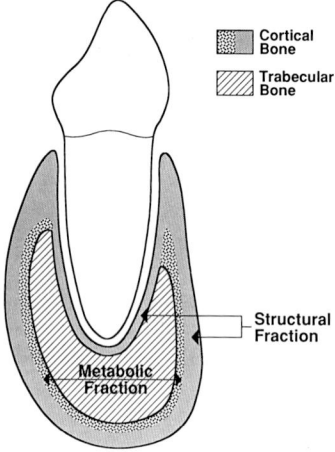

Cortical Bone

Trabecular Bone

Structural Fraction

Metabolic Fraction

Fig. 1. Metabolic and structural fractions of alveolar and basilar bone. The structural fraction is controlled by biomechanical factors (functional loads, etc.). The metabolic fraction is a reservoir of calcium to meet metabolic needs. (From *Roberts* et al., Implant Dentistry in preparation).

fourth power of its diameter. By a similar mechanism of focussed bone resorption and formation events, trabeculae can form, reorient and change in size as a result of "micromodelling" to resist functional loads optimally[2]. A good example of this process (Fig. 3) is the network of secondary trusses that forms in the marrow cavity to support an integrated fixture.[10]

Cortical bone remodelling (internal turnover) is accomplished by paravascular cutting/filling cones, a functional unit of the osteoclasts and osteoblasts organized around a proliferating, dedicated blood vessel (Fig. 4). Trabecular bone (spongiosa) remodels in a similar manner, by means of "hemi-cutting/filling cones" that selectively remove and replace a set volume of bone at specific foci (Fig. 5). The main difference in trabecular remodelling is the lack of an internal, dedicated blood supply. The hemi-cutting/filling cone depends on the vascularity of the marrow.

Trabecular bone remodels at a rate of 20–30% per year. From a metabolic perspec-

tive, spongiosa is the most important calcium reserve in the body[5, 6]. Virtually all trabecular bone is within the metabolic fraction. Remodelling can be accomplished without compromising structural integrity because, first, only a small portion of the supporting osseous tissue is turning over at any one time and, secondly, the remodelling process preferentially affects the metabolic fraction, structurally the least important bone[13].

Under most circumstances, cortical bone remodels at a rate of about 2–10% per year. Since only a portion of the cortex is in the metabolic fraction, the remodelling rate for cortical bone is usually 3–10 times less than for adjacent trabecular bone (metabolic fraction)[6]. At a few localized sites, such as the alveolar process, the temporomandibular joint, and the interface of osseointegrated implants, cortical bone turnover is ≥ 30% per year[11]. This elevated remodelling rate is probably related to the high stress and subsequent fatigue damage caused by masticatory function. Thus,

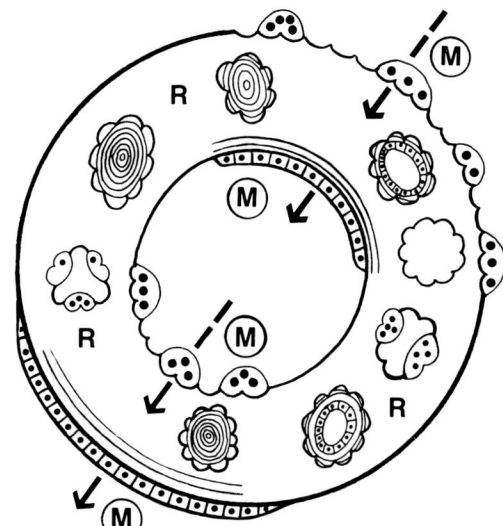

Fig. 2. Modelling (M) represents a series of uncoupled formation and resorption events that change the size, shape or position of a bone. Remodelling (R) is the turnover of previously existing bone. Modelling (M) is largely controlled by functional loading, while remodelling responds primarily to demand for metabolic (ionic) calcium[9].

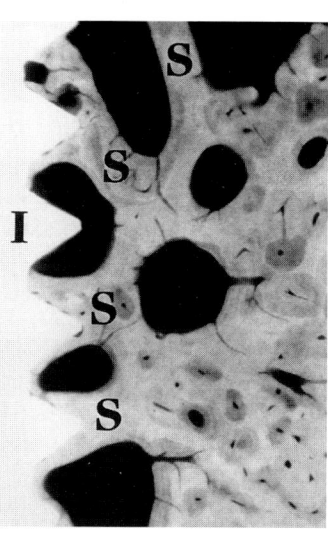

Fig. 3. Osseous adaptation to a rigidly integrated fixture involves formation of new secondary trabeculae (S) to support functional loading. Adapted from *Roberts* et al.[10]

the most critical bone in the dental apparatus is highly labile and susceptible to mechanical overload.

Calcium metabolism

Calcium metabolism is vital to life. About 99% of body calcium is in bone, in effect, the skeletal system serves as a metabolic reservoir (Fig. 6). When challenged by sustained negative calcium balance (low calcium diet, oestrogen deficiency, long-term corticosteroid treatment, etc.), the least mechanically protected portions of the skeleton are preferentially resorbed.[5] Metabolically compromised edentulous and partially edentulous patients are particularly susceptible to loss of jaw structure. Not only is the alveolar process resorbed, but there is also extensive loss of bone from the

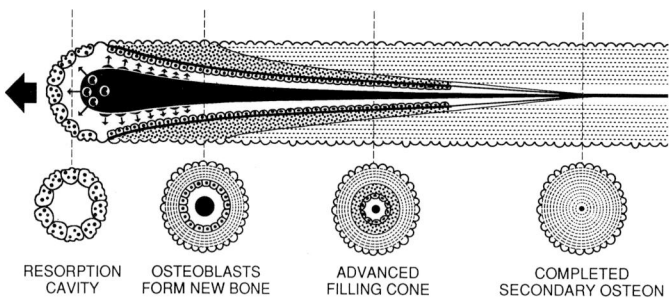

Fig. 4. The cutting/filling cone is the mechanism of cortical bone remodelling (turnover). The cutting head of osteoclasts, derived from circulating precursor cells, removes old bone. The trailing filling cone of osteoblasts, derived from paravascular cells, forms a new secondary osteon. Adapted from *Roberts* et al.[13]

RESORPTION CAVITY   OSTEOBLASTS FORM NEW BONE   ADVANCED FILLING CONE   COMPLETED SECONDARY OSTEON

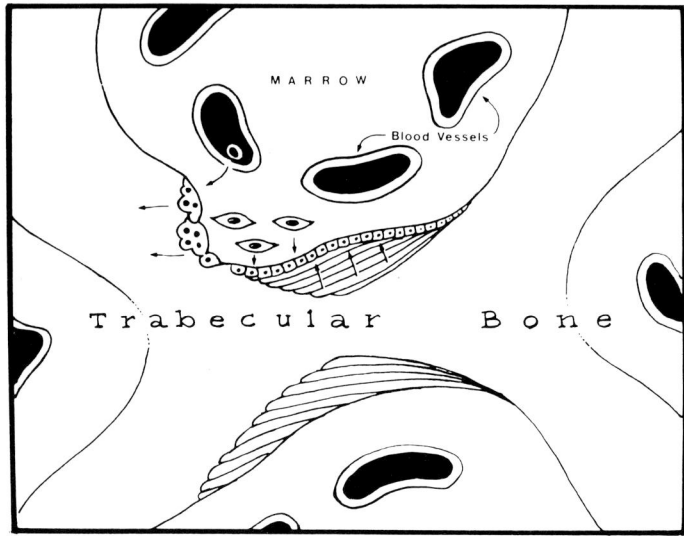

Fig. 5. The hemi-cutting/filling cone is the mechanism of trabecular bone remodelling. It is similar to the cutting/filling cone of cortical bone except that it has no internal vascular supply and must depend on the blood supply of the adjacent marrow.

metabolic fraction, i.e. trabecular bone and the inner (endosteal) portion of the cortex. In individuals with optimal oral function, similar metabolic demand tends to spare the jaws and preferentially mobilizes calcium from other parts of the body (Fig. 7a, b, c).

Metabolic bone disease

An evaluation of bone metabolism is a key element in diagnosis. The screening procedure must involve a careful medical history, evaluation of signs and symptoms of skeletal disease, and an assessment of risk factors associated with negative calcium balance[13]. The most prevalent metabolic bone diseases in middle-aged and older patients are:

(1) Paget's disease: a malignancy affecting the osteoclasts and resulting in localized resorption cavities filled with immature woven bone (irregular radiolucencies on radiographs);

(2) Renal osteodystrophy: poor bone

CALCIUM METABOLISM

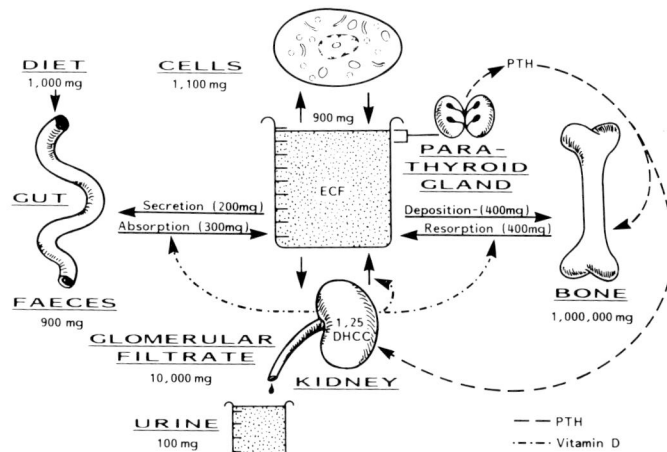

Fig. 6. Calcium metabolism to maintain bone mass (zero calcium balance)[13].

quality secondary to inadequate kidney function (also referred to as fibrous dysplasia);

(3) Hyperparathyroidism: elevated serum calcium is often associated with high turnover osteopenia (low bone mass) secondary to a parathyroid adenoma;

(4) Thyrotoxicosis (hyperthyroidism or overtreatment of hypothyroidism): high turnover osteopenia;

(5) Osteomalacia: poor mineralization of osteoid due to a deficiency of the active metabolite of vitamin D (1.25 dihydroxycholecalciferol);

(6) Osteoporosis: symptomatic osteopenia, usually resulting in fractures of the spine, wrist and/or hip.

Osteopenic risk factors

Patient with a negative calcium balance are a poor risk for oral implant procedures because of progressive skeletal atrophy. Risk factors for low skeletal mass (osteopenia or "osteoporosis") are:

(1) age: progressive incidence in older patients;

(2) race: white caucasians and asians from industrialized countries are preferentially affected;

(3) sex: females are predominantly affected;

(4) genetics: there is a strong familial tendency;

(5) slight stature: particularly when maintained by habitual dieting;

(6) diet: calcium deficient and/or excessively high protein (meat) consumption;

(7) exercise: lack of consistent, strenuous activity;

(8) tobacco: osteopenia is directly related to the amount of nicotine consumed;

(9) alcohol: related to excessive consumption, defined as more than about ten oz/week;

(10) pharmaceuticals: corticosteroids, lithium, anticonvulsants (Dilantin™, etc.), thyroid hormone and a number of other long-term drug regimens[8].

161

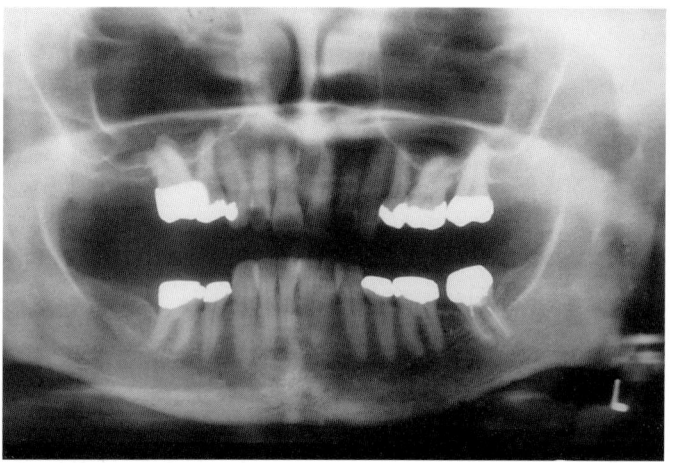

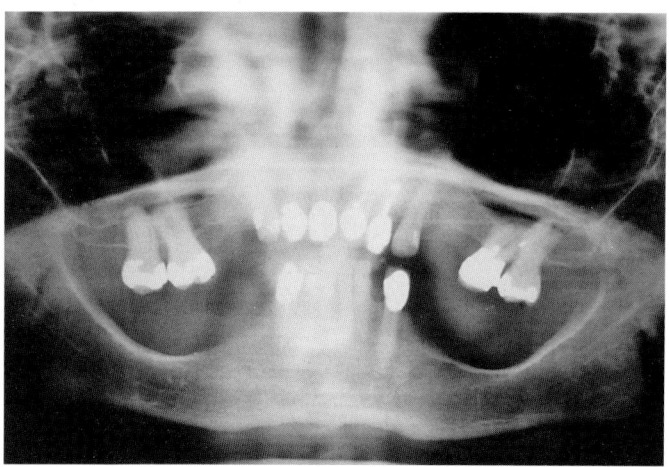

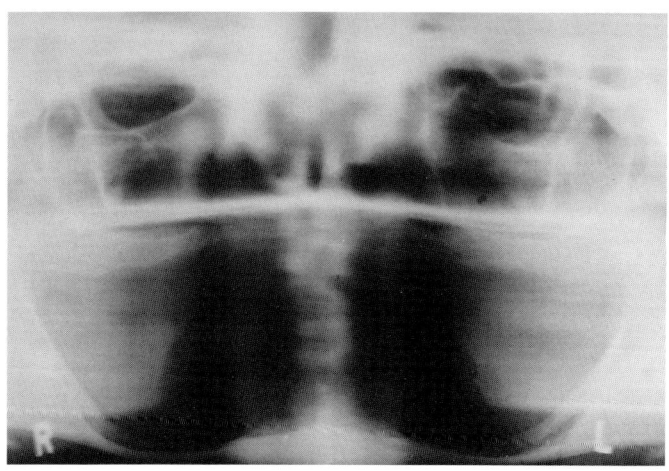

Fig. 7. Dental panoramic radiography of three postmenopausal females showing varying degrees of osteopenia. (a) When key teeth are preserved in all four quadrants, functional loads protect the bone from metabolic resorption. (b) Loss of the lower posterior teeth results in disuse atrophy of the alveolar process. (c) Severe resorption is due to edentulousness· (poor mechanical loading) and negative calcium balance secondary to long-term, low dose corticosteroid therapy. From *Roberts* et al. (in preparation).

Therapeutic measures

Although remodelling is essentially a physiological mechanism for repairing fatigue damage and providing metabolic calcium, the rate of turnover must be controlled. Under steady state conditions, remodelling is accomplished at a structural cost. Each ARF cycle results in a slight negative calcium balance, i.e. not quite as much bone is replaced as was removed. A normal rate of remodelling results in a slow, age-related loss of bone (senile osteopenia). Within limits; this physiological loss of bone is not a problem, because structural demands diminish with age. However, an excessive rate of bone remodelling, such as is seen in postmenopausal women or in cases of thyrotoxicosis, may result in high turnover osteopenia or osteoporosis[6].

From a metabolic perspective, the remodelling rate (number of ARF events/unit time) is enhanced by both parathyroid (PTH) and thyroid (TH) hormones. PTH is a specific hormone for mobilizing and conserving calcium primarily within the metabolic fraction (Fig. 1). TH increases remodelling by elevating the metabolic rate of the entire body. Oestrogen suppresses the remodelling rate; for this reason oestrogen replacement therapy (ERT) is very effective in preventing the high turnover osteopenia characteristic of the menopause. Growth hormone (GH) and anabolic steroids (AS) also tend to build skeletal mass, but by a completely different mechanism. They enhance muscle mass which stimulates periosteal bone formation (modelling) to build the structural fraction of bone. Despite their well established anabolic effects, neither GH nor AS is commonly used to treat osteoporosis, because of side-effects such as cardiac hypertrophy and other acromegalic signs[13]. Metabolic bone disease is a complex medical problem that should be treated by specially trained physicians with access to appropriate diagnostic and treatment monitoring equipment. Such facilities are available in most major medical centres, usually associated with the Endocrinology Section of the Department of Internal Medicine. Depending on the aetiology, osteopenia or osteoporosis may be treated with exercise, dietary supplements (calcium and/or vitamin D), hormones and/or specific drugs. Bone loss may be suppressed by decreasing the remodelling frequency with oestrogen (ERT) or by directly inhibiting resorption with calcitonin or bisphosphonates. ERT is usually considered to be the most effective long-term therapy for women. At present there is no equivalent hormonal therapy for men[13].

Oestrogen treatment is no problem for prospective oral implant patients. However, calcitonin, bisphosphonates and other antiresorptive drugs can cause problems, because bone resorption is an essential element for post-operative healing and long-term maintenance of integrated implants. Devitalized, immature and fatigued bone can only be removed by osteoclastic activity.

Bone loading

Bone cells are sensitive to strain (deformation) along functionally loaded bone surfaces. The peak strain history of dynamic (normal cyclic) loading is related to the magnitude and frequency of functional loads. From published data and clinical experience, *Frost*[3] has proposed a biomechanical relationship for skeletal adaptation; referred to as the "mechanostat." The strain-mediated hierarchy of bone atrophy, maintenance, hypertrophy, and pathological overload is well accepted, but the actual strains which control these events may be site-specific (Fig. 8).

Bone is a composite biomaterial that structurally adapts to its mechanical environment. It is well suited to a lifetime of function when optimally loaded within the physiological range. Suboptimal loading results in atrophy of both bone mass and structural orientation. The upper limit of the physiological loading range for steady-state maintenance of bone is only about 10% of its ultimate strength (2500/25000 microstrain, μE). Moderate overloading (10–15% of ultimate strength) induces a hypertrophic response to increase bone mass and optimize structural orientation. Pathological overload (>16% of ultimate strength) is defined as repeated (cyclic) loads exceeding the usual adaptive capacity of the bone. Accumulation of fatigue damage may result in localized loss of osseous support (bone recession, craters, etc.) or a spontaneous stress fracture[4].

Mechanical loading optimizes mineralized tissue mass, quality and orientation. An extensive alveolar process supports the teeth in both jaws. Because the maxilla is loaded primarily in compression, its osseous structure is similar to the body of a vertebra, i.e. predominantly trabecular bone with thin cortical plates. In the maxilla, the palatal plate is generally thicker than the labial plate. The mandible has much thicker cortices than the maxilla because it acts as a cantilever, and is subjected to substantial torsion (Fig. 9a).

Alveolar bone, the specialized osseous tissue that is formed to support teeth, probably requires a higher strain to avoid atrophy than does the basilar bone of the jaws. When teeth are lost, the alveolar process often resorbs until only the basilar mandible and maxilla remain (Fig. 9b). Rigid bone implants restore atrophic bone to masticatory function (Fig. 9c). Prostheses

supported by osseointegrated implants present unique biomechanical challenges because of:

(1) the extended "crown – root ratio" of the suprastructure;
(2) the lack of a cushioning periodontal ligament (PDL);
(3) the compromised neurological feedback mechanisms for controlling occlusal force.

All of these factors tend to concentrate the occlusal load at the periosteal margin of the supporting bone. Heavy functional loads and/or poor prosthetic load distribution can contribute to failure of the implants, its suprastructure and/or adjacent bone through fatigue. Clinicians must be particularly vigilant in avoiding mechanical overloading during the first year of function. The osseous support is fragile because of the high rate of turnover and lack of mineral maturation[9].

Bone tissue

Three distinct types of bone (woven, lamellar and composite) are involved in implant integration, i.e. post-operative healing and maturation. Woven bone is highly cellular, has a rapid formation rate (30–50 μm/day or more), a relatively low mineral density, more random fibre orientation, and poor strength. Since woven bone is more compliant than mature osseous tissue, it plays an important stabilizing role in the initial healing of endosseous implants. Although capable of stabilizing an unloaded implant, woven bone lacks the strength to resist masticatory forces. Lamellar bone is the principal load-bearing tissue of the adult skeleton. It is the predominant component of a mature bone/implant interface (Fig. 10). Lamellar bone is formed relatively slowly (<1.0

Dynamic Loading

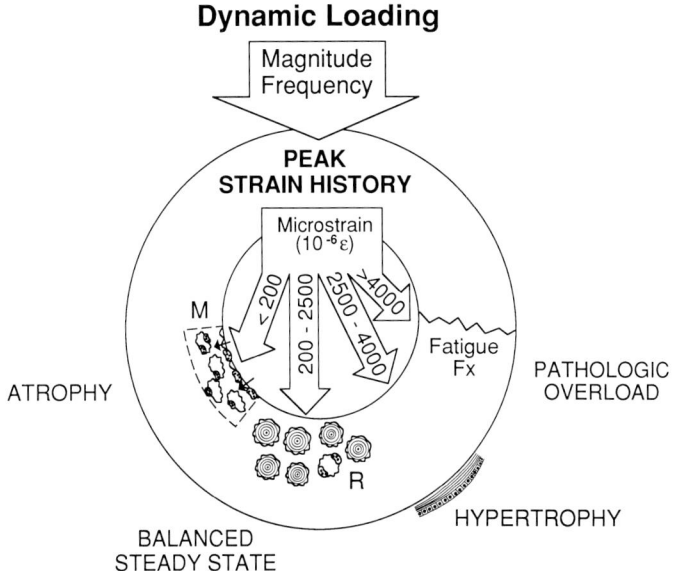

Fig. 8. Biomechanical control of osseous adaptation (bone modelling and remodelling) is related to the magnitude and frequency of dynamic (intermittent) loads. The peak strain history (bone deformation over time) dictates the osseous response. Bone deformation (strain) is expressed as microstrain (μE) which is strain x 10^{-6}. Since per cent strain is 10^{-2}, 1000 μE is the same as 0.1 per cent strain. Repetitive loading at more than 4000 μm results in pathological overload and eventual fatigue failure of bone. From *Roberts* et al. (in preparation).

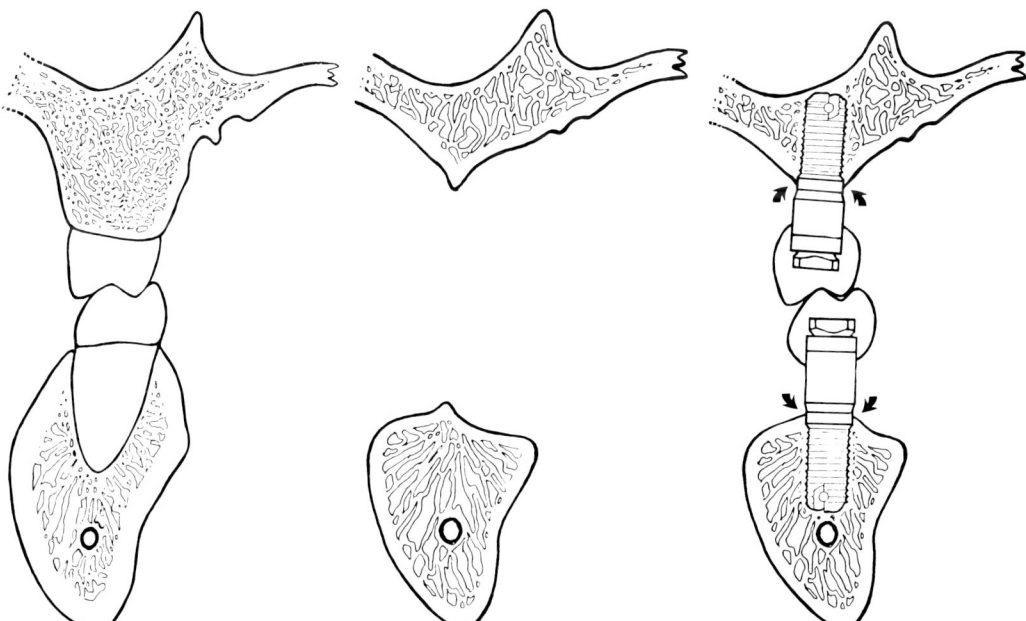

Fig. 9. (a) When natural teeth have normal bone support, there is a relatively short lever arm from occlusion to the level of alveolar bone. (b) Resorption of the edentulous alveolar process increases the vertical dimension between the maxilla and mandible. (c) Implant-supported prostheses constitute a long lever arm from occlusal contact to the level of bone support. Thus, lateral forces in occlusion place a heavy load on bone where the alveolar crest contacts the implant.

165

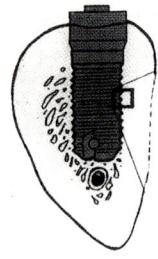

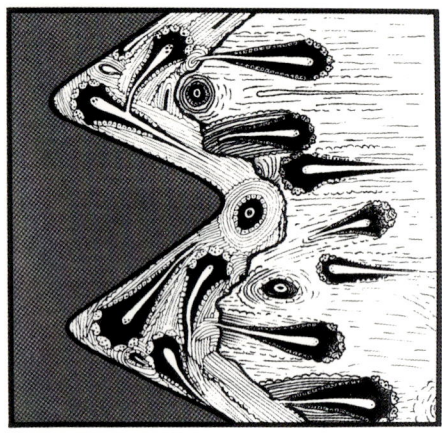

Fig. 10. Schematic drawing showing the dynamic healing and maturation sequence for a bone implant. Numerous cutting heads (osteoclasts) and filling cones (osteoblasts) remodel the interface and supporting bone. From Roberts et al. (in preparation).

µm/day), has a highly organized matrix and is densely mineralized. Composite bone is a combination of paravascular lamellar bone deposited on a woven bone matrix. During the initial wound healing phase, a highly porous, woven bone lattice (callus) emanates from intact (unstripped) periosteum at the periphery of the wound. The highly vascular callus grows towards the implant on both the endosteal and periosteal surfaces. The paravascular cavities then fill with high quality lamellae, thus gaining adequate strength for load bearing[7]. Formation of composite bone is an important step in the stabilization of an implant during the rigid integration process.

Implant integration

The cortical bone response to an integrated implant involves five physiological stages:

(1) Callus formation: initial, cytokine-driven response to stabilize the fixture (0.5 months);
(2) Callus maturation: lamellar compaction, remodelling, and reduction of the callus (0.5–1.5 months);
(3) Regional acceleratory phenomenon (RAP): remodelling of the non-vital interface and supporting bone (1.5–12 months);
(4) Maturation of osseous integration: completion of the RAP, secondary mineralization of new bone and increased direct bone contact at the interface (4–12 months);
(5) Long-term maintenance of osseointegration: continuous, localized remodelling events to repair fatigue damage within interfacial and supporting bone (>12 months)[11].

Prior to the installation of implants, most edentulous sites are atrophic as a result of inadequate mechanical loading. Placing an oral implant overrides the atrophic mechanism and elicits a time-dependent, localized healing response that is controlled primarily by local cytokines from the blood clot and adjacent injured tissue. The post-operative acceleration of bone remodelling (RAP) lasts for about a year (3 sigma). During the first 4 months (1 sigma), the major events are:

(1) Resolution of post-operative inflammation;

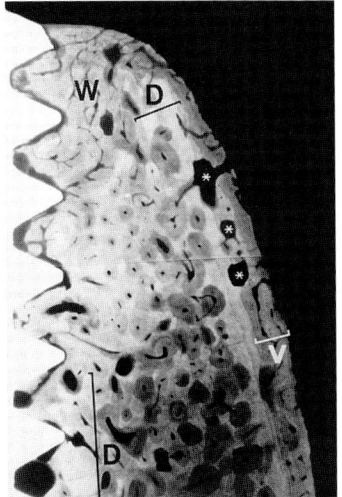

Fig. 11. Microradiograph of a bone fixture in dog mandible displaying modelling and remodelling activity associated with 2 months of unloaded healing followed by a 4-month loaded phase. Woven bone (W) can be seen at the alveolar crest. Devitalized areas (D) are seen where the periosteum was stripped and bone was tapped at the time the implant was placed. New vital bone (V) has formed on the devitalized layer during the subsequent healing phase. Intense remodelling (white stars) has occurred in the subperiosteal layer of devitalized bone[9].

(2) Callus formation and maturation;

(3) Initiation of bone remodelling at the interface and within supporting bone (Fig. 10). After about a 4-month closed healing phase in cortical bone (6 months in trabecular bone), the implant should be uncovered and subjected to progressive functional loading. It is important to begin loading at about 4–6 months, to take advantage of the bone mass generated by the healing process. If not optimally loaded, the newly formed bone will atrophy. As the healing response subsides, mechanical and metabolic factors re-establish control of bone structure. Bone generated by the cytokine-driven healing response will only be retained if it is adequately loaded[14].

Despite severe loss of bone structure, a compromised patient may still experience a normal healing response. However, if mechanical and metabolic deficiencies are not corrected, the negative physiological environment will persist after the healing response subsides. This is likely to be detrimental to the maturation and long-term maintenance of implant-supported prostheses.

Progressive loading

The healing and maturation phases of implant integration are dependent on modelling and remodelling (Fig. 11). Maturation of the mineralized interface and supporting bone is a critical step in the integration process. There is a direct relationship between age of bone and its mineral density. Following a maturation phase of about one week, newly formed osteoid is mineralized by a large number of small hydroxyapatite crystals. During this period of primary mineralization, osteoblasts deposit about 70% of the mineral found in mature vital bone. Secondary mineralization (the remaining 30%) is a noncellular crystal growth phenomenon that occurs over a period of about 8 months (Fig. 12). Mineral maturation is important to integrated implant support, because the stiffness and strength of lamellar bone is directly related to its mineral content[1].

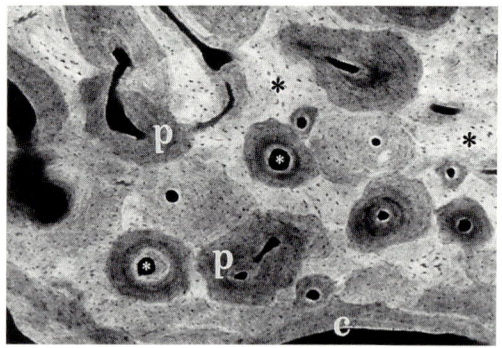

Fig. 12. A microradiograph of compact bone near an integrated implant shows bone with varying degrees of mineralization due to modelling and remodelling. New circumferential lamellae (C) are seen at the periosteal surface. New bone displaying primary mineralization (P) is visible in the more radiolucent osteons. As the new osteons age, gradients of secondary mineralization (white stars) increase mineral content and the rigidity of the osseous tissue. Mature, fully mineralized bone is marked with black stars.

Failure of immature bone in supporting osseointegrated implants is a common clinical problem during the first year of masticatory function. To provide an optimal mechanical environment during the first 6–9 months after restoration of masticatory function, progressive loading is recommended:

(1) Utilize a rigid suprastructure to avoid flexure and optimize implant loading;
(2) Progress from a soft to hard diet over a period of 6 months;
(3) Guard against parafunctional habits (clenching, bruxism, etc.).

Long-term maintenance of osseointegration

Long-term maintenance of a rigid implant interface is related to continual bone remodelling. Occasionally, successfully integrated implants are removed for orthodontic and/or prosthetic purposes. Two doses of tetracycline (7–10 days apart) immediately prior to implant removal will provide important dynamic information on the steady-state remodelling associated with maintenance of osseointegration. From a series of double-labelled implants in func-

tion for 3 years or more, it appears that maintenance of a viable bone – implant interface requires continual remodelling activity at a relatively high rate ($\geq$ 30% turnover per year)[11]. Preferentially replacing the oldest bone first, the process of remodelling continuously renews interfacial and supporting bone by repairing foci of fatigue damage while maintaining the overall structural integrity of the integrated device. The specialized remodelling process, within about 1 mm of the implant surface, is apparently the mechanism for maintenance of osseointegration (Fig. 13).

Management of severely resorbed jaws

Spontaneous fractures are common when bones become fragile due to reduced bone mass, loss of trabecular connectivity and accumulation of fatigue damage (Fig. 14). Bone continues to atrophy in an unfavourable metabolic and/or mechanical environment[5]. Long-term edentulousness in the presence of a negative calcium balance is commonly associated with a severe and progressive atrophy of the jaws. Patients with atrophy of the jaws present a substan-

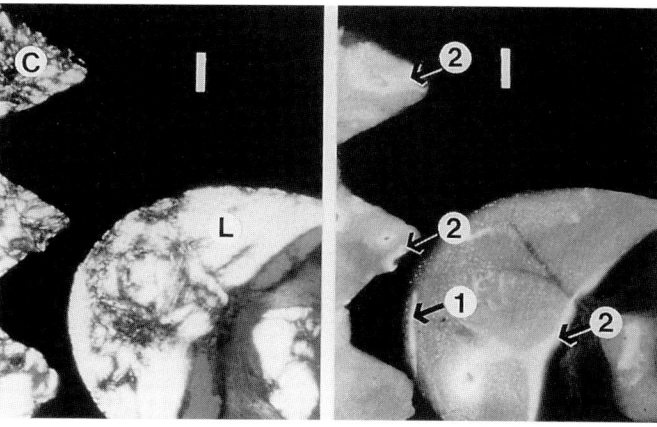

Fig. 13. Polarized light (left) and UV fluorescence (right) 100 μm sections demonstrate mature lamellar bone in the threads (C) and in the apical hole through the implant (L). This fixture was utilized for orthodontic anchorage in the mandibular retromolar area for about 3 years. The first (1) and second (2) fluorescent bone labels, administered prior to removing the implant, demonstrate a high rate of bone remodelling within 1 mm of the bone–implant interface.[11]

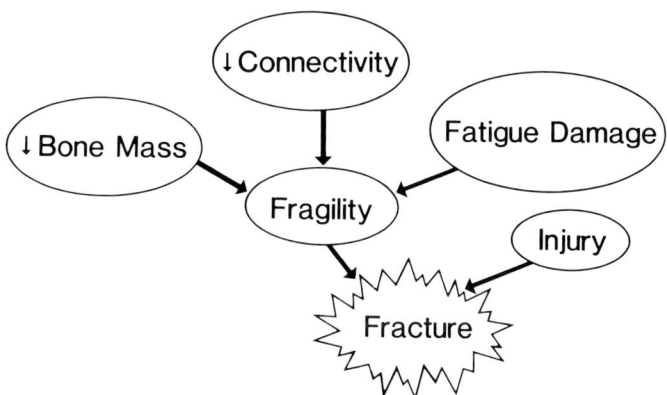

Fig. 14. Factors contributing to bone fragility. Adapted from *Roberts* et al.[12]

tial clinical challenge, but can still be treated with integrated implants if:

(1) The negative calcium balance is corrected;

(2) Adequate skeletal mass remains; and/or

(3) Osseous structure can be restored with bone grafts.

It is important to realize that even fragile bones have a strong healing potential. The problem in treating patients with low bone mass is not a healing deficiency, but lack of structural reserve to resist the post-operative weakening which is characteristic of the bone healing process.[14] Weakening a severely atrophic mandible by drilling holes to install implants may result in a spontaneous fracture within a few weeks. Despite this distressing complication, the bone will heal if adequately stabilized. Assuming sufficient implants are retained or re-installed, a successful prosthetic restoration is possible.

Summary

Skeletal compromise is the rule rather than the exception for edentulous and partially edentulous patients. Rigid integrated implants represent a range of new treatment possibilities, provided that the clinician appreciates the complexity of the integration process with respect to host compatibility. Routine clinical success with rigid (osseointegrated) bone implants demands a firm grasp of the modern concepts of bone physiology, metabolism and biomechanics.

References

[1] *Currey, J. D.* The mechanical adaptations of bones. pp. 1–294. Princeton: Princeton University Press, 1984.

[2] *Frost, H. M.* Intermediary organization of the skeleton. Volume 1, pp. 1–365. Boca Raton: CRC Press, 1986.

[3] *Frost, H. M.* Some ABCs of skeletal pathophysiology. 6. The growth/modelling/remodelling distinction. Calcif Tissue Int 1991; *49:* 301–302.

[4] *Martin, R. B., Burr, D. B.* Structure, function, and adaptation of compact bone. pp. 1–275. New York: Raven Press, 1989.

[5] *Midgett, R. J., Shaye, R., Fruge, J. F.* The effect of altered bone metabolism on orthodontic tooth movement. Am J Orthod 1981; *80:* 256–262.

[6] *Parfitt, A. M.* The physiological and clinical significance of bone histomorphometric data. In: *Recker, R. R.* (ed.). Bone histomorphometry: Techniques and interpretation. pp. 143–223. Boca Raton: CRC Press, 1983.

[7] *Roberts, W. E.* Bone tissue interface. J Dent Educ 1988; *52: 804–809.*

[8] *Roberts, W. E., Garetto, L. P., Arbuckle, G. R., Simmons, K. E., De Castro, R. A.* Bone physiology: evaluation of bone metabolism. J Am Dent Assoc 1991; *122:* 59–61.

[9] *Roberts, W. E., Garetto, L. P., De Castro, R. A.* Remodelling of devitalized bone threatens periosteal margin integrity of endosseous titanium implants with threaded or smooth surfaces: Indications for provisional loading and axially directed occlusion. J Indiana Dent Assoc 1989; *68:* 19–24.

[10] *Roberts, W. E., Helm, F. R., Marshall, K. J., Gongloff, R. K.* Rigid endosseous implants for orthodontic and orthopedic anchorage. Angle Orthod 1989; *59:* 247–256.

[11] *Roberts, W. E., Marshall, K. J., Mosary, P. G.* Rigid endosseous implant utilized as anchorage to protract molars and close an atrophic extraction site. Angle Orthod 1990; *60:* 135–152.

[12] *Albrektsson, T., Lekholm, U.* Osseointegration: Current state of the art. Dent Clin of North America, 1989; 531–554.

[13] *Roberts, W. E., Simmons, K. E., Garetto, L. P., De Castro, R. A.* Bone physiology and metabolism in dental implantology: Risk factors for osteoporosis and other metabolic bone diseases. Implant Dent 1992; *1:* 11–21.

[14] *Roberts, W. E., Smith, R. K., Zilberman, Y., Mozsary, P. G., Smith, R. S.* Osseous adaptation to continuous loading of rigid endosseous implants. Am J Orthod 1984; *86:* 95–111.

Chapter 9

Tissue response to loading and microbiota

M. Quirynen

Clinical parameters for the evaluation of soft and hard tissues

Although differences exist in the composition of the periodontium around teeth and implants, the clinical parameters for the evaluation of the health of soft and hard tissues are identical. It is, however, important to relate the values of these parameters to the specific periodontal situation.

In the natural dentition, the periodontium comprises the soft tissue (gingiva and/or alveolar mucosa), the periodontal ligament, the root cementum and the jaw bone. For osseointegrated implants; both root cementum and periodontal ligaments are absent. Just as around teeth, the soft tissue around healthy implants establishes a cuff-like barrier which adheres to the surface. For both types of abutment, the epithelial cells adhere to the surfaces by means of hemidesmosomes. However, because of the absence of root cementum around implants, the orientation of the collagen fibres in the connective tissue differs. Around teeth, the fibre bundles run "perpendicular" to the root cementum, but around implants these fibres, which begin at the marginal bone, are oriented "parallel" to the metal surface[1].

These fibres, although not imbedded in the implant surface, form a seal which is strong enough to arrest epithelial downgrowth, thereby preventing epithelial encapsulation, also known as marsupialization. The importance of the absence of a periodontal ligament was discussed in Chapters 5 and 7.

Over the years, several measuring methods have been used to determine the extent of periodontal destruction around teeth. Pocket probing and radiographic bone examination are still the most accurate and commonly used methods in clinical practice. The value of these techniques in the follow-up of implants will be discussed first.

Attachment level

For teeth as well as for implants, the probing pocket depth (PPD: the distance from the gingival margin to the bottom of the pocket; Fig. 1) is a meaningful clinical parameter in the long-term evaluation of the periodontium. Around implants, however, the "initial" probing pocket depth in fact only reflects the thickness of the surrounding mucoperiosteum; which might be 7 mm or more. Thus, by itself, probing pocket depth does

171

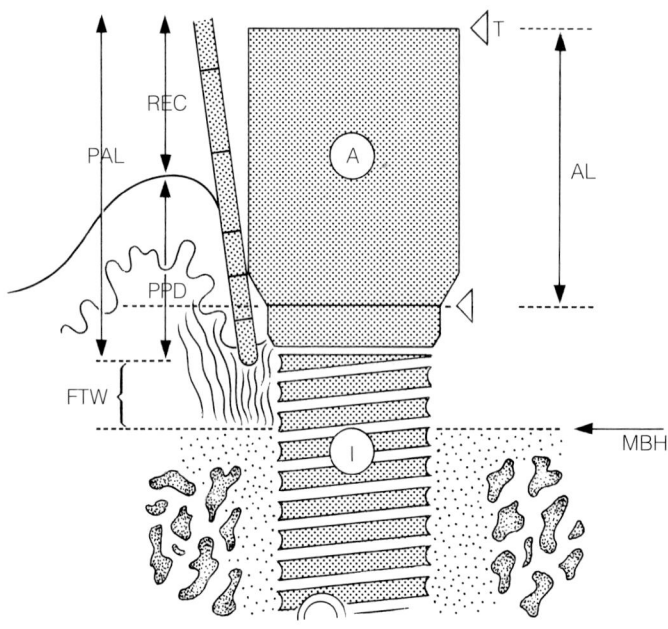

Fig. 1. Schematic representation of clinical parameters. A (abutment): extends through the mucoperiosteum, making the connection between implant and prosthetic reconstruction; I (implant): inserted in the bone; T (top of the abutment): junction between abutment and prosthetic superstructure; IAJ (implant/abutment junction): reference level for bone loss measurement; REC (recession): distance from the top of the abutment to the marginal border of the soft tissue; PPD (probing pocket depth): distance between the marginal border of the soft tissue and the tip of the pocket probe; PAL (probing attachment level): distance between the top of the abutment and the tip of the pocket probe (PAL = REC+PPD); FTW: width of the fibrous tissue; AL: abutment length; MBH: marginal bone height.

not give much information; in fact, it depends on the surgeon, who often has the opportunity to trim the mucoperiosteal flap, thereby reducing the pocket depth. Only a "change" in depth should attract attention. In this respect, it is important to remember that the location of the gingival margin also often changes with time. Particularly in cases where a removable denture is replaced by a fixed implant-supported prosthesis, apical migration of the gingival margin may occur. Therefore, the gingival recession (REC: the distance from the top of the abutment to the gingival margin; Fig. 1) should also be measured. The sum of the PPD and the REC represents the probing attachment level (PAL; Fig. 1) which is defined as the distance from the top of the abutment to the bottom of the pocket. This parameter, which takes into consideration both the pocket depth and the location of

the gingival margin, is the most meaningful parameter. An increase in this distance often indicates a loss of supporting bone. Moreover, the probing attachment level offers the possibility of calculating the position of the tip of the periodontal probe in relation to the implant. If the PAL is larger than the abutment length, the probe has penetrated apically to the implant/abutment junction. If it is smaller, the probe has remained coronal to this junction. The probing attachment level should be measured at 6-month intervals. For each implant, six locations should be probed: mesiobuccal, mid-buccal, distobuccal, mesiolingual, mid-lingual and distolingual). Special attention should be paid to keep the probe exactly parallel to the long axis of the abutment. Sometimes the design of the prosthetic reconstruction does not allow reproducible measurement of the PPD. In

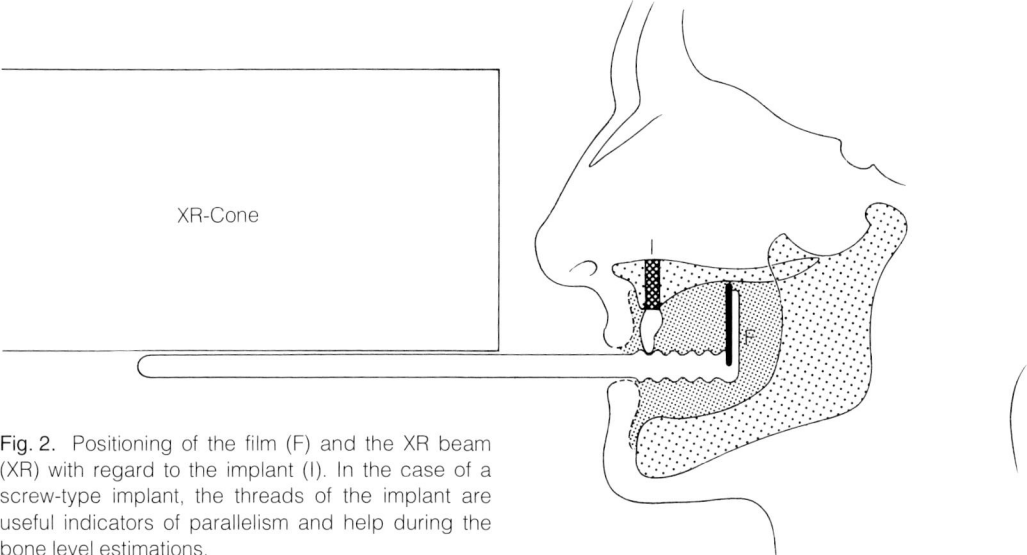

Fig. 2. Positioning of the film (F) and the XR beam (XR) with regard to the implant (I). In the case of a screw-type implant, the threads of the implant are useful indicators of parallelism and help during the bone level estimations.

such cases, only reproducible sites per implant should be considered. As for the natural dentition, an increase of 2 mm or more in probing attachment level should be interpreted as a loss in supporting tissue.

It does appear that pocket probing around implants is more painful than around natural teeth. Whether this reflects histological differences in the soft tissue between teeth and implants is not yet well understood. Preliminary studies also indicate that the use of a constant probe pressure does not necessarily increase the reproducibility of pocket probing around implants.

Radiographic bone level estimation

Optimal intra-oral radiographs can provide valid information about the health of peri-implant tissues. For oral implants, as for teeth, the use of a long-cone, parallel technique and intra-orally placed films is indispensable. The parallel technique is illustrated in Fig. 2. The film is positioned orthoradially to the implant, with the longer edges parallel to the implant's longitudinal axis. The XR beam direction must be perpendicular to this axis. A film holder should be used to obtain this position and to increase the reproducibility of the technique. Good reproducibility is of the utmost importance, since a comparison between radiographs at time intervals offers the most useful clinical information (Fig. 3). High quality images can be obtained only if a long cone XR beam is used (Fig. 3). Due to the radiopacity of most implants, radiographs – in contrast to probing – only give information about the approximal area. The

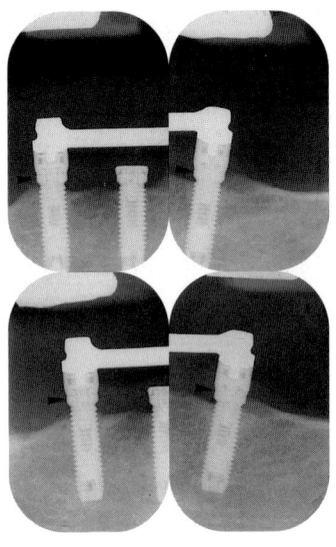

Fig. 3. Consecutive radiographs (4 months and 3 years after denture installation) showing screw-type implants supporting an overdenture. The two lateral implants are interconnected by means of a straight bar to which the denture is anchored. The implant in the middle, a sleeping implant, can be used in case of implant loss. Both loaded implants showed minor bone loss during the first 6 months of loading (upper radiographs) but from then on the bone level remained stable. The implant/abutment junction is arrowed.

bone level both mesially and distally can be measured by means of a calliper. It must not be forgotten, however, that infra-bony pockets are not always visible on radiographs, so that more bone loss may sometimes be present than can be seen on the radiograph. This explains why a combination of radiographic examination and pocket probing is advocated.

Radiographs may show a peri-implant radiolucency, indicating a loss of osseointegration. In a normal follow-up protocol, radiographs should be taken at 3-year intervals or whenever complications occur.

In severely resorbed lower jaws, in particular, attempts at imaging the entire length of the implant may cause discomfort and even pain to the patient. However, relaxation of the muscles of the floor of the mouth and of the tongue (mylohyoid, geniohyoid, and genioglossus muscles), will facilitate the examination. In most cases, however, the peri-implant tissue can be adequately assessed even if the apical part is omitted.

Relationship between the probing attachment level and the bone level

Because radiographic examination should not be repeated too frequently, to avoid undue radiation exposure, the only means of regular clinical examination is pocket probing. Fortunately, there is a good correlation between the bone level estimated from radiographs and the tip of the pocket probe (probing attachment level). For Brånemark (screw type) implants, the mean marginal bone level was scored 1.2 mm apically of the probing attachment level; for IMZ (plasma-sprayed) implants, this distance (called fibrous tissue width [FTW] in Fig. 1) was 1.1 mm.[2] If a significant loss of attachment, recorded by probing, does not correspond to the radiographic image, an infra-bony defect may be present. In such cases, a radiograph taken with a gutta percha point or a periodontal probe in the pocket can offer more information.

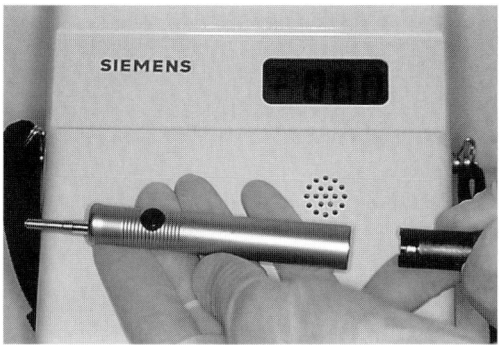

Fig. 4a. The Periotest TM apparatus, consisting of a microcomputer and handpiece.

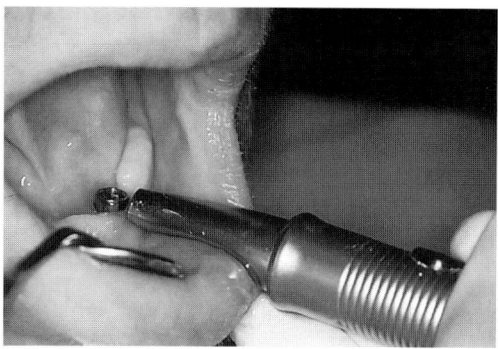

Fig. 4b. Percussion using the Periotest TM device just below the edge of the coronal platform of the abutment.

Mobility

In contrast to the natural dentition, immobility is an essential parameter for osseointegrated implants. In teeth, the degree of mobility does not correlate with the quality and/or quantity of the supporting tissue. Indeed, a tooth with a healthy and unreduced periodontium but with a traumatic occlusion, can demonstrate a very high degree of mobility, whereas a tooth with a 50% reduced but healthy supporting tissue may still be scored as immobile. Osseointegrated implants should not show any clinical mobility; the slightest increase in mobility indicates the development of a problem.

In the clinic, only crude indices are available to examine the mobility of implants. However, an electronic device, the Periotest™ (Siemens AG, Bensheim, Germany) gives an objective estimation of implant mobility. The equipment consists of a microcomputerized measuring and steering device, connected to a handpiece (Fig. 4). The handpiece incorporates a rod (8 g), which is accelerated forwards by touching a start button. The rod moves forward at almost constant speed until it hits the implant. After impact, the implant is deflected and the rod is braked. The reaction forces bring the implant back to its original position and the rod is reaccelerated, back into the starting position. This cycle is repeated so that, over a period of 4 seconds, 16 defined, reproducible impacts with the implant are obtained. A miniature accelerometer at the end of the rod sends signals to the microcomputer, which calculates the braking time. The final Periotest value (PTV) ranges from -8 to $+50$. A braking time of 346 microseconds corresponds to a PTV of -5, whereas a braking time of 466 microseconds gives a PTV score of $+2$. Thus, the firmer the abutment the lower the PTV score. For healthy, monoradicular teeth the PTV varies from $+1.5$ to $+7$. A score of less than $+10$ indicates a clinically immobile situation, while with scores of $+10$ or more, mobility may

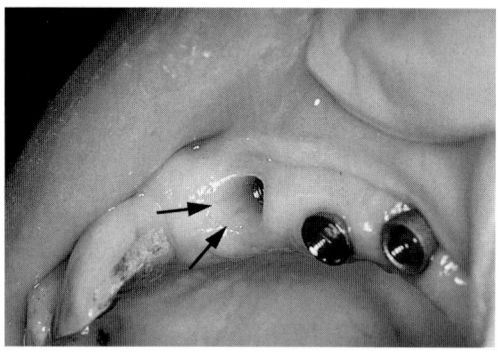

Fig. 5. In this patient with an implant-supported partial prosthesis in the anterior region, the bridge was removed in order to examine implant mobility. After removal of the permucosal part, the soft tissue wall around the implant is visible. The arrows indicate soft tissue lesions, corresponding to probing locations.

be clinically detected. A score of +30 represents mobility which might be caused by lip or tongue pressure.

For healthy implants the PTV score ranges from +5 to −8, with a mean score of about −1[3]. The score will depend on implant size (the larger the implant, the lower the score), the abutment length (the smaller the abutment, the lower the score), and the bone quality (more negative scores in the more compact lower jaw). For implants with a PTV score of more than +5 an extended clinical investigation is recommended, including measurement of the PPD and the bone level, and with a check-up of oral hygiene, gingival inflammation, and occlusion and articulation. If a score of +10 to +15 is obtained, loss of osseointegration should be diagnosed and the implant should be removed before abscesses form.

In order to examine the mobility of an implant, it is, of course, essential to remove the fixed prosthesis. However, frequent removal of the fixed prosthesis is not recommended, because replacement may initiate increased stress on the implants. Implant mobility should only be scored when the prosthesis is removed in the event of complications or at 5-year intervals.

Bleeding on probing and gingivitis indices

The prognostic value of bleeding on probing and other gingivitis indices is not yet well understood. The differences in the histology of the soft tissues around implants may be reflected in these parameters. Fig. 5 shows an approximal soft tissue wall around an implant with a healthy gingiva, after pocket probing and abutment removal. The vertical lesions correspond to the location of probing.

Microbiota around implants

Plaque formation on oral implants is still an almost unexplored topic, especially since, compared to the natural dentition, additional variables complicate the story. Several studies clearly illustrate that the surface characteristics of implants significantly affect bacterial adhesion. Clear positive correlations have been reported between surface roughness and the rate of bacterial recolonization, both supra- and subgingivally.

Unfortunately, in several implant systems, the part which penetrates the mucosa and/or extends supragingivally is extremely rough. Also, the surface free energy (the energy available on a surface to attract a liquid) was found to have a significant influence on the amount and composition of the adhering bacteria. Surfaces with a lower surface free energy seemed to harbour less plaque with less pathogenic bacteria. Since these parameters may differ from one implant system to another, it is almost impossible to draw final conclusions, or to extrapolate data from one implant system to another.

It is, however, important to make a clear distinction between the partial and fully edentulous situation. Clinical studies report significantly fewer integrating implants in patients with severe and untreated periodontitis of the remaining natural dentition, a phenomenon which may be explained by direct (saliva) or indirect (bloodstream) contamination. Other investigators have clearly proved that, in partial edentulism, the pockets around the remaining teeth act as a reservoir for the colonization and recolonization of the implants. These observations, indicate the importance of an optimal periodontal health in the natural dentition prior to implant installation. Moreover, fully edentulous patients, especially those with a longer period of edentulism prior to implant insertion, spontaneously lose some important periodontal pathogens such as *Porphyromonas gingivalis* and it may take some time before they become re-infected after implant insertion.

Soft tissue response to loading and microbiota

Immediately after abutment installation, an initial change in the soft tissue may be observed. Due to a healing process of this tissue following elimination of the traumatic effect of a removable denture, a shrinkage of up to 2 mm often occurs over a period of 3 months. Therefore, the final decisions concerning abutment length and prosthesis design should be postponed until the end of this period. Meanwhile, a provisional, but rigid, prosthesis, attached to all the implants, should prevent individual loading of the latter and should offer considerable comfort to the patient. The long-term measurement of probing pocket depth has only been reported for Brånemark implants. In this system, a small reduction in PPD with time has been recorded, together with a comparable increase in gingival recession, indicating a relatively stable probing attachment level. In rare cases with an increased PPD, radiographic examination showed local bone loss.

The reaction of the periodontium around teeth and Brånemark implants to supragingival plaque formation has been studied in an animal model. Both tissue reactions were shown to be identical, with a comparable increase in leukocyte transmigration and a comparable apical extension of connective tissue infiltration for both abutments.

In the presence of an overdenture, a proliferation of the gingiva around implants may sometimes occur. This is mostly the result of denture-induced trauma and/or poor oral hygiene. Stringent oral hygiene, good denture design, and the removal of the denture at night are key factors in the maintenance of a healthy mucosa.

As with teeth, the presence of gingivae around implants does not appear to be a prerequisite for maintaining gingival health. However, in some rare cases with alveolar mucosa around implants, food impaction in the pocket can lead to local infection and exposure of the threads (in the case of a screw-type implant) and may lead to trauma. Such complications are rare, and do not justify the unrestricted use of free gingival grafts.

Hard tissue response to loading and microbiota

The widely accepted criteria for successful oral implants[4] include the absence of any peri-implant radiolucency and an annual vertical bone loss of less than 0.2 mm following the implant's first year of service. Due to bone remodelling after abutment and prosthesis installation, early bone loss around the implants often occurs. Some months after loading, the bone should reach a stable level, which often corresponds to the most coronal thread in the case of a screw-type implant or the specially prepared surface in the case of a cylindrical implant[5]. From then on, bone level should remain stable. Sleeping implants show hardly any bone loss. The unchanged bone level around these implants may be explained by the absence of loading, thus avoiding overstressing of the marginal bone (at least in the case of screw-type implants) which results in mechanical breakdown of the bone[5].

It must also be born in mind that the quality of the osseointegration increases with time. In an animal study[6], Johansson and Albrektsson reported an increase in the area of direct contact between implant and surrounding bone until 1 year after insertion. Moreover, the torque levels necessary for implant removal increased significantly over this period, from 10 to 88 Ncm. This indicates that osseointegration is a "living" process and continues to develop over time. It is therefore important to increase the loading of newly installed prostheses slowly. Patients should be instructed to masticate extremely carefully, at least during the early months following rehabilitation. This increase in the level of osseointegration is also reflected in increased stability when examined by means of a Periotest™ (more negative score).

In addition to implant type and host response (see Chapters 5.2 and 5.3) other factors also influence long-term bone stability around osseointegrated implants. These include implant design, prosthetic reconstruction, occlusal load, and oral hygiene.

Minor changes in the design of an implant greatly influence the clinical outcom[7]. In addition, occlusal overload (due to a lack of anterior contact in case of a cantilever bridge, the presence of parafunctional activity, and/or the presence of an osseointegrated full fixed prosthesis in the opposing jaw) may lead to excessive marginal bone loss around osseointegrated implants[8]. These parameters should, therefore, receive special attention. In patients with parafunctional habits for example, more implants and/or a night guard might be indicated in order to control the overload.

The relationship between marginal bone loss around osseointegrated implants and subgingival plaque is not yet well understood, owing to the contradictory results in animal studies as compared to in vivo studies. Lindhe et al.[9] compared the effects of ligature-induced periodontitis around teeth and implants in beagles. They observed that ligature placement around implants resulted in an inflammatory process which, as in the case of teeth, resulted in marginal bone loss. However, with implants, the extent of the inflammatory lesion was more pronounced, with more bone loss and a larger area of infiltrated connective tissue. The investigators suggested that this difference was related to differences in the infection and/or the local host response.

The most conspicuous difference between the lesions around implants and teeth was the extension of the connective tissue infiltrate, which reached the bone crest in the case of implants in four out of five dogs. Sometimes it even extended into the bone marrow. However, one might question whether the ligature model is suitable for this kind of study, since for the same implant system previous animal experiments [10–11] – with experimental gingivitis, but without ligatures – did not report such dramatic bone losses. Perhaps the resistance of the peri-implant soft tissue, without imbedded collagen fibres (they run parallel to the surface), is insufficient for this applied "unnatural" trauma.

The interpretation of in vivo studies is even more complicated. In deep pockets around implants with considerable bone loss the flora is comparable to that detected around periodontally involved teeth. It is characterized by a larger proportion of Gram-negative anaerobic rods (e.g. black-pigmented Bacteroides and Fusobacterium species) and an increased concentration of spirochaetes. However, the question remains whether these organisms induced the bone loss or whether they simply found ideal growing conditions in pockets which had been created by overloading. It is clear that more research is needed in this area before final conclusions can be drawn. However, one should remember that long-term clinical studies, unfortunately only available for the Brånemark system, clearly illustrate that in patients with good oral hygiene, osseointegration can last for 20 years or more.

References

[1] Van Drie, H. J. Y., Beertsen, W., Grevers, A. Healing of the gingiva following instalment of Biotes implants in beagle dogs. Adv Biomater 1988; 8: 485–490.

[2] Quirynen, M., Naert, I., van Steenberghe, D., Duchateau, L., Darius, P. Periodontal aspects of Brånemark and IMZ implants supporting overdentures: A comparative study. In: Laney, W. R., Tolman, D. E. (eds). Tissue integration in oral, orthopedic and maxillofacial reconstruction. pp. 80–93. Chicago: Quintessence Publishing Co., 1992.

[3] Teerlinck, J., Quirynen, M., Darius, P., van Steenberghe, D. Periotest TM: An objective clinical diagnosis of bone apposition toward implants. Int J Oral Maxillofac Implants 1991; 6: 55–61.

[4] Albrektsson, T., Zarb, G., Worthington, P., Eriksson, R. A: The long-term efficacy of currently used dental implants: a review and proposed criteria of success. Int J Oral Maxillofac Implants 1986; 1: 11–25.

[5] Pilliar, R. M., Deporter, D. A., Watson, P. A., Valiquette, N. Dental implant design – Effect on bone remodelling. J Biomed Mater Res 1991; 25: 467–483.

[6] Johansson, C., Albrektsson, T. Integration of screw implants in the rabbit: A 1-year follow-up of removal torque of titanium implants. Int J Oral Maxillofac Implants 1987; 2: 69–75.

[7] Quirynen, M., Naert, I., van Steenberghe, D., Schepers, E., Calberson, L., Theuniers, G., Ghyselen, J., De Mars, G. The cumulative failure rate of the Brånemark™ system in the overdenture, the fixed partial, and fixed full prostheses design: a prospective study on 1273 fixtures. J Head Neck Pathol 1991; 10: 43–53.

[8] Quirynen, M., Naert, I., van Steenberghe, D. Fixture design and overload influence marginal bone loss and fixture success in the Brånemark system. Clin Oral Implant Res 1992; 3: 104–111.

9 *Lindhe, J., Berglundh, T., Ericsson, I., Liljenberg, B., Marinello, C.* Experimental breakdown of peri-implant and periodontal tissues. A study in the beagle dog. Clin Oral Implant Res 1992; *3:* 9–16.

10 *Brånemark, P.-I., Breine, U., Adell, R., Hansson, B.* O., Lindström, J., Ohlsson, Å. Intra-osseous anchorage of dental prostheses. I Experimental studies. Scand J Plast Reconstr Surg 1969; *3:* 81–100.

11 *Klinge, B.* Implants in relation to natural teeth. J Clin Periodontol 1991; *18:* 482–487.

Chapter 10

Complications and failures

Ph. Worthington

Success and failure

Various concepts of success and failure with oral implants have evolved over the years. It is now generally accepted that in order to be regarded as "successful", an endosseous implant must do more than just remain in the jaw[1]. It must also demonstrate clinical immobility, even under load-bearing conditions. The implant should be free from associated symptoms such as discomfort, pain and tenderness. There should be no impairment of function of adjacent structures, such as the inferior alveolar nerve and its mental branch, and there should be no progressive, continuing radiolucency surrounding the implant. Loss of crestal bone height should be minimal (Table I).

Table I. Endosseous implants: criteria for success

Clinical immobility
Ability to bear load
No associated symptoms
No damage to adjacent structures
No progressive peri-implant radiolucency
Minimal loss of crestal bone height

In order to avoid failure, patients must be carefully selected, not only to ensure favourable anatomical features and the absence of diseases of the jaw bone, but also that they have no unreasonable expectations about the outcome. Meticulous, thoughtful planning is fundamental to success, as is full discussion between the surgeon, the restorative dentist and the patient. The surgeon must adhere to a strict surgical protocol and the prosthetic device must be carefully designed and accurately constructed. Finally, careful maintenance is important to the longevity of the reconstruction. Under these desirable conditions, osseointegration may be anticipated in a high proportion of cases. When failures do occur, they are usually, but not always, attributable to deviation from the abovementioned principles; patient selection may have been imprudent, planning may have been faulty, consultation between clinicians may have been inadequate, or there may have been faults in technique during the surgical, prosthetic and laboratory phases of treatment.

Osseointegration may fail to develop or, having developed, may later be lost. We do not always know the cause of failed osseointegration. In some instances, it may be a "biological" failure, for example where blood supply to the bone is poor or where the bone is inadequate in quantity, quality or density. It may be an "iatrogenic" failure, as when bone is overheated during implant site preparation. Osseointegration may subsequently be lost due to overloading, perhaps as a consequence of poor prosthetic design, casting inaccuracy or the patient's parafunctional habits.

Indications of failure

Persistent tenderness associated with an implant is a bad omen. When the patient says "one implant just does not feel right" one should be on the lookout for failed osseointegration.

Mobility of an endosseous implant is a clear sign of failure and such an implant should be removed. However, the clinician must be able to distinguish between the mobility of an incompletely attached abutment and the mobility in the underlying implant itself.

The development of a radiolucent line around an implant on a radiograph is not usually an early sign of failure, but, where present, indicates that the bone has receded from the implant surface and the intervening space is occupied by granulation tissue or a fibrous tissue sheath.

When an individual implant fails, the clinician will remove it and may allow the site to heal completely before attempting to replace the failed implant with a new one. Under special circumstances, some clinicians will clean the implant site of granulation and fibrous tissue and will attempt immediate replacement with an implant of greater diameter.

Complications

Complications may result from biological, iatrogenic or mechanical factors. Examples of biological factors which produce complications include bone of poor quality or inadequate volume, smoking, previous irradiation or immunosuppression.

Iatrogenic factors include inappropriate case selection, faulty planning, deviation from the recommended surgical protocol and prosthodontic overloading due to poor design.

Mechanical factors play a part when manipulation is heavy-handed or when a patient exhibits parafunctional habits such as bruxism.

Serious complications

Since the placement of oral implants is an elective procedure, it may seem strange that some complications have been so serious as to cause fatalities. Death from air embolism has resulted from the mistaken use of a coolant spray of compressed air and water with internally irrigated drills[2]. This can also cause serious surgical emphysema. It cannot be too strongly emphasized that practitioners must not deviate from the manufacturers' recommendations regarding the equipment to use and the means of using it. Such tragedies are avoidable.

Life-threatening haemorrhage has been reported as a result of instrument perforation of the lingual cortex of the mandible during implant site preparation, with damage to small vessels in the floor of the mouth[3, 4]. Bleeding may then progress into the soft tissues of the floor of the mouth causing a threat to the patient's airway, and necessitating emergency surgical treatment. Careful surgery, exploration of lingual con-

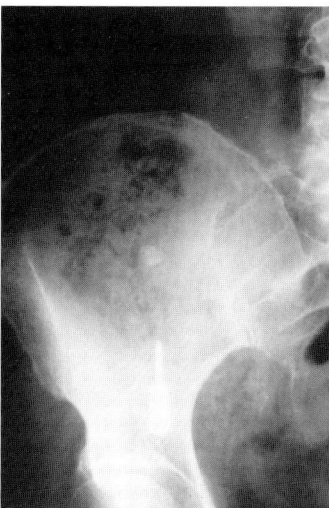

Fig. 1. Radiograph shows a small screwdriver lodged in the patient's pelvis; its progress was arrested at the ileo-caecal junction. The instrument was later removed successfully by fibreoptic colonoscopy.

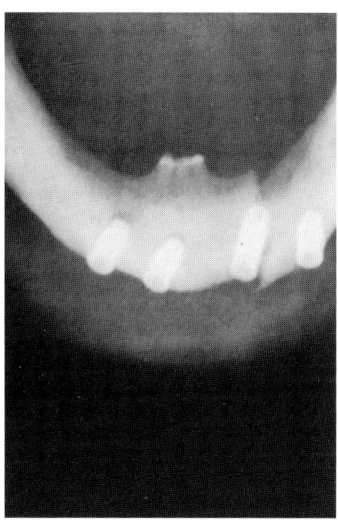

Fig. 2. Radiograph showing fracture of the mandible through the site of an endosseous cylinder implant.

cavities at operation and post-operative patient supervision are necessary.

Many implant components are small, as are the instruments involved. When coated with saliva they may escape from the clinician's grip and fall into the oropharynx, where reflex swallowing may take the item out of sight almost instantly. This is a particular risk in the recumbent patient. The item may thus be ingested or, even worse, inhaled. If this should happen, the patient should be immediately placed in a head down position and an attempt made to recover the lost component. If it has gone too far, the patient should be transported to a hospital in a head-low position, so that the appropriate endoscopy can be carried out (Fig. 1).

Fracture of the atrophic mandible has been reported in several instances and will certainly have occurred in many unreported cases[5]. This emphasizes the need for great care in patient evaluation, in surgery and in after-care. Patients with an atrophic mandible must be warned to take great care during the post-operative period. The treatment of a fractured atrophic mandible is never easy, but when the jaw bone contains several recently placed, expensive implants that occupy space that might otherwise be used for plates and screws, the situation is even more critical (Fig. 2).

Damage to the inferior alveolar nerve has been reported due to misplaced implants; this indicates the need for detailed planning, including, in some cases, specialized presurgical radiographic assessment by computerized tomography (Fig. 3).

Complications associated with implant placement

Faulty implant placement may take several forms. Implants may be placed too close together, so that it is difficult to attach the abutments, or to keep the intervening mucosa healthy. They may be placed too far to

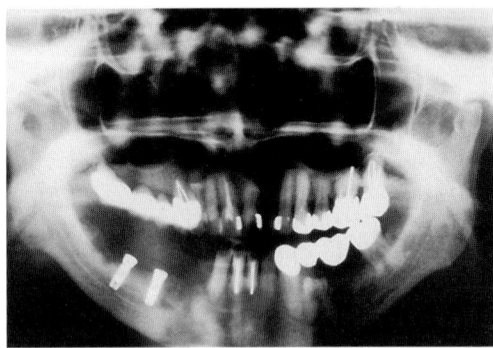

Fig. 3a. Panoramic tomogram indicating probable intrusion of implants into the inferior alveolar nerve canal.

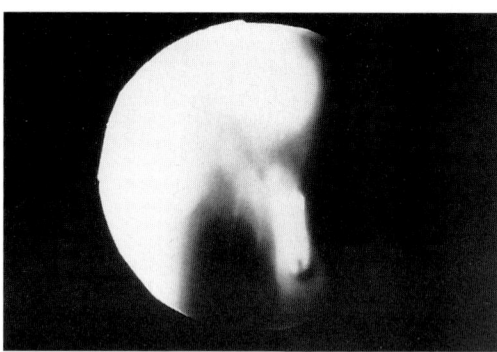

Fig. 3b. This tomogram confirms the penetration of an endosseous implant into the inferior alveolar canal; this resulted in loss of sensation in the region of the mental nerve.

the labial or buccal aspect of the jaw, resulting in exposure of the implant as the site is enlarged (Fig. 4). With care this undesirable situation may be remedied by the placement of bone grafts over the exposed surface or by the use of so-called guided tissue regeneration techniques using special membranes. Similarly, implants placed too far lingual may be at risk owing to the thin, vulnerable and mobile mucosa of the floor of the mouth. Faulty angulation of implants may be avoided by care in planning and by the use of templates to guide the surgeon, and can sometimes by remedied by the use of angulated abutments.

Excessive countersinking at the mouth of the implant site is to be avoided, especially in the posterior region of the mandible, where internal support for the implant may be lacking due to the loosely textured trabecular bone.

If the drill is damaged or eccentric, or badly handled, the resultant implant site may be ovoid in cross-section instead of circular. Implant–bone contact will therefore be diminished, with a consequent lessening of the

chances of successful osseointegration. When bone is overheated during the preparation of the implant site, bone cells in the immediate vicinity of the interface have less chance of surviving. The bone may "die back" from the implant surface, to be replaced by less differentiated scar tissue; this heralds failure. Thermal damage to the bone must therefore be avoided by the use of sharp drills, intermittent and gentle pressure, drills of incremental sizes, copious coolant irrigation and strictly controlled rotational drill speeds.

Dehiscence of the incision may occur if there is premature loading of the recently operated site (e.g. by the premature wearing of a denture), or if the denture is inadequately relieved over the implant sites. Breakdown of the wound is particularly likely to occur if there has been previous irradiation of the area or even previous surgery (such as a visor osteotomy or the placement and removal of a subperiosteal implant). These factors all tend to impair the blood supply to the area and extra precautions must be taken (Fig. 5).

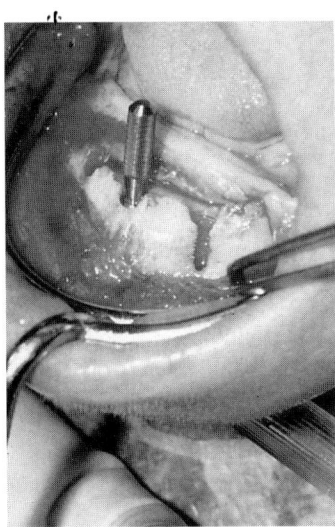

Fig. 4. Labial placement of this implant resulted in exposure of the threads on the labial aspect. Had a template been used, this error might have been avoided.

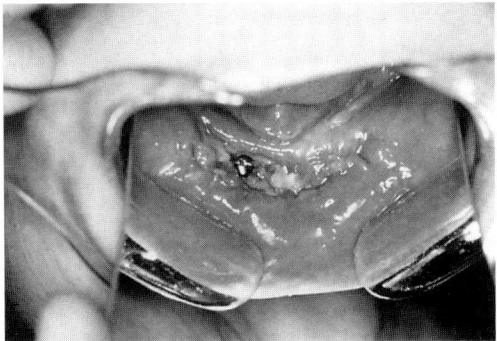

Fig. 5. Dehiscence of the incision used for implant placement. This was attributed to previous irradiation of the area during treatment of an oral carcinoma.

Complications associated with abutment connection

It is sometimes difficult to judge with accuracy the desirable height of the abutments at the time of placement; it may be necessary to change the abutments later, or, alternatively, to use so-called healing abutments temporarily, until the peri-implant soft tissue has settled down and stabilized.

The seating of the abutment cylinder on the implant must be accurate. Many systems have interlocking hexagonal projections and recesses and if the abutment cylinder is incompletely seated, this may result in soft tissue hyperplasia, infection and possible fistula formation (Fig. 6).

Complications associated with the restorative and maintenance phases

Abutment screws, may loosen during construction of the prosthetic device, and should be checked periodically to see that they are tight.

Casting the base of the prosthesis requires great skill on the part of the laboratory technician. A base that does not fit absolutely passively will cause unequal distribution of forces and may lead to serious problems. Complications seen during the prosthetic and maintenance phases include breakage of the abutment screws or gold screws and, occasionally, fracture of the cast base (Fig. 7). When acrylic material is used to provide the occlusal surface of the prosthesis, this may split and break off if it is not thick enough.

Poor oral hygiene tends to produce gingivitis and gingival hyperplasia.

Where a maxillary implant prosthesis has a space between the base plate and the alveolar crest, there may be an initial problem with air escaping during speech; in the short term, this can be corrected by fitting a removable dam in the form of a gingival veneer, but the patient usually undergoes a

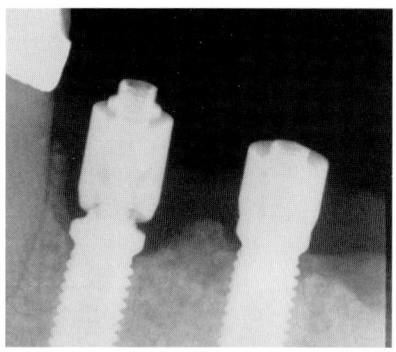

Fig. 6. Note that one of the abutments in this radiograph is incompletely seated. This should be connected before treatment continues.

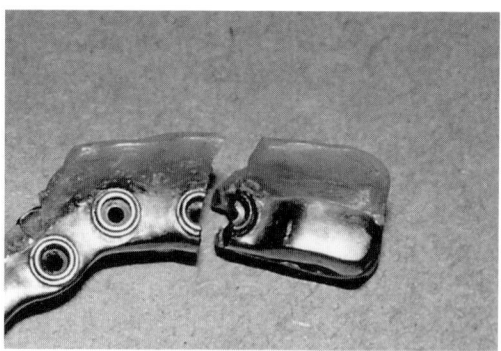

Fig. 7. Fracture of the whole prosthesis, including the metal baseplate. The cross-sectional design of the baseplate casting is important, as is the length of the cantilever extension.

process of adaptation and, after a period, the veneer no longer seems to be necessary.

Summary

All implant systems have their history of problems and complications[6, 7]. These can usually be avoided by attention to detail during patient selection, patient care, planning, the clinical stages, and the maintenance phase. Intelligent anticipation will allow many problems to be avoided altogether. Careful follow-up can lead to early detection of incipient complications. With reputable implant systems, the problems and complications that do occur are usually due to deviation from the recommended protocol and should occur less frequently as experience is gained.

Complications deserve our most serious attention, not merely because of the effect on the patient, but because the reputation of implant dentistry as a whole is at stake. We need to exercise the greatest care throughout the whole treatment period; small errors in planning or technique may cause greatly magnified effects in the end result.

References

[1] Albrektsson, T., Zarb, G., Worthington, P., Eriksson, A. R. The long term efficacy of currently used dental implants: a review and proposed criteria of success. Int J Oral Maxillofac Imp 1986; 1: 11–25.

[2] Davies, J. M., Campbell, L. A. Fatal air embolism during dental implant surgery: report of three cases. Can J Anaesth 1990; 37: 112–121.

[3] Mason, M. E., Triplett, R. G., Alfonso, W. F. Life-threatening hemorrhage from placement of a dental implant. J Oral Maxillofac Surg 1990; 48: 201–204.

[4] Laboda, G. Life-threatening hemorrhage after the placement of an endosseous implant: report of a case. J Am Dent Assoc 1990; 121: 599–600.

[5] Mason, M. E., Triplett, R. G., van Sickels, J. E., Parel, S. M. Mandibular fractures through endosseous cylinder implants: report of cases and review. J Oral Maxillofac Surg 1990; 8: 311–317.

[6] Worthington, P., Bolender, C. L., Taylor, T. D. The Swedish system of osseointegrated implants: problems and complications encountered during a 4-year trial period. Int J Oral Maxillofac Imp 1987; 2: 77–84.

[7] Worthington, P. Problems and complications with osseointegrated implants. In: Worthington, P., Brånemark P.-I. (eds). Advanced osseointegration surgery: applications in the maxillofacial region. Chicago: Quintessence Publ. Co., 1992.

Chapter 11

Maxillofacial reconstruction

J. F. Tulasne

Reconstruction of the facial skeleton is best achieved with autogenous bone grafts protected by local or regional flaps. Over the past decade, maxillofacial reconstruction has stimulated new interest because of the application of new surgical procedures and new devices such as osseointegrated implants.

Indications

Indications for bone reconstruction and oral rehabilitation are the same; whatever the cause of the anomaly. The only exceptions are patients who have previously been irradiated, since such patients have reduced healing capacities and therefore need special care. Indications vary according to the localization and size of the bone defect. The timing of treatment also depends on the extent of the anomaly.

Treatment planning

It is generally preferable to follow the rule "first to build, then to place the implants". Planning the oral rehabilitation in two or three stages is certainly safer for achieving an ideal result, both morphologically (vol-

ume of the graft) and functionally (position of implants and final dental occlusion).

However, simultaneous placement of the implants and the bone graft can be considered in the case of a partial defect, where a sufficient amount of basal bone and some remaining teeth can provide a strong anchorage and ideal positioning of the implants through the graft.

Size of the bone defect

Small defects can be treated by a graft taken either from the chin or from the iliac crest. Large and irregular defects of the maxilla are best corrected using a large piece of iliac bone, which can easily be contoured to fit the defect exactly. Missing parts of the mandible are reconstructed with either a cranial or an iliac graft. Cranial grafts are the ideal material to reinforce a thin and high alveolar crest.

Location of the bone defect

The maxilla

The reconstruction of large defects in the maxilla is often made difficult by oronasal or

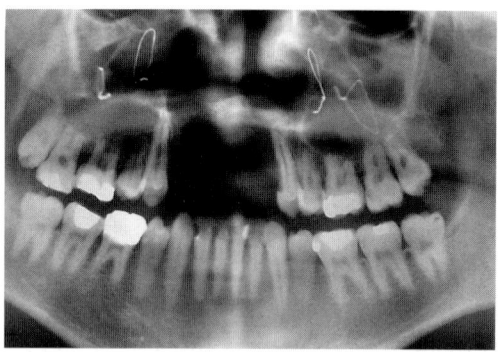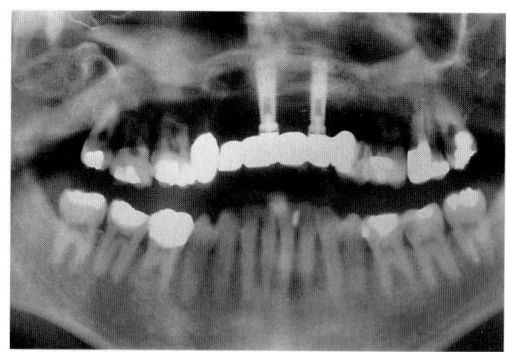

Fig. 1. (a) Secondary deformities of a bilateral cleft lip and palate in a 22-year-old patient who previously had 24 operations. The premaxilla is totally missing, and there is a large oronasal fistula. Reconstruction was performed in three stages (*Tessier* and *Tulasne*).
(b) Condition of the patient at the end of the treatment, with cranial grafts and two Brånemark implants in place. (Courtesy of Cahiers de Prothèse, № 71, Septembre 1990.)

oro-antral fistulae. This problem can be solved by using a temporalis muscle flap which fills the maxillary sinus and provides a partition between the nasal and oral cavities (Fig. 1a and b). When closure of the mucosa is possible, either on the nasal or the oral side of the fistula, an osteo-muscular flap can be used, and the bone fragment will serve as a basis for the future construction of the maxilla.

The mandible

Mandibular reconstruction (Fig. 2a and b) for continuity defects requires perfect immobilization of the bone segments. Intermaxillary fixation is often unreliable, as many teeth may be missing. Strong osteosynthesis plates (macroplates) are invaluable in stabilizing the fragments and the bone graft rigidly. In irradiated patients, the graft is wrapped in temporalis muscle; or some type of vascularized bone graft may be considered.

Vestibuloplasty

Reconstruction of the jaws often results in loss of the vestibule, which may make maintenance of good oral hygiene extremely difficult. A vestibuloplasty is often indicated, with a gingival or split skin graft. It can be performed before or after abutment connection.

Principles of bone reconstruction

Some basic principles must be respected in order to ensure the long-term success of a bone graft. These are related to the area to be grafted (recipient site), the shape and volume of the graft and the soft tissues covering the graft. They are not specific to the maxillofacial area.

(1) The recipient site must be perfectly "freshened" and sufficiently large to ensure revascularization of the graft. Any remnant of soft tissue or poorly vascularized bone is removed by burring the bone until the area to be grafted is bleeding.

In maxillary and mandibular reconstruction, the teeth adjacent to the recipient site

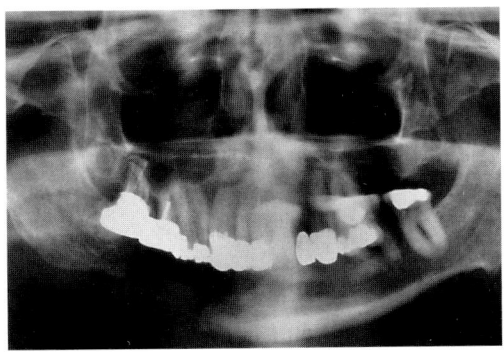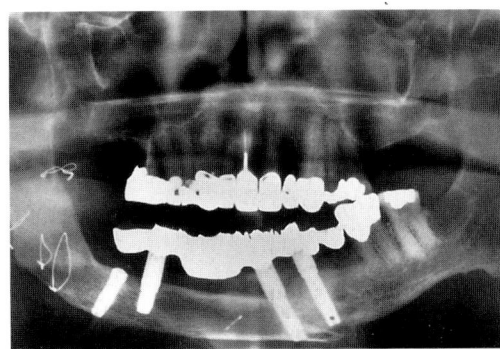

Fig. 2. (a) Patient with post-traumatic loss of part of the right mandible (war injury). Several attempts at reconstruction were unsuccessful. The patient also had radiotherapy for a carcinoma of the lower lip.
(b) Reconstruction was performed in several stages, including cutaneous flaps, iliac and cranial grafts, and implants (*Tessier* and *Tulasne*). A fixed bridge was constructed (*G. Hure*).

should be extracted unless they are perfectly healthy.

(2) The graft must fit the recipient site as closely as possible. It should be contoured to fill the bone defect and to have a large contact surface with the area or the bone fragments to be grafted. Any dead space will inevitably result in haematoma formation and possible infection; or the development of fibrous tissue.

The volume of the graft must be carefully evaluated. There is a limit to the amount of bone that can be expected to "take" as a free graft at any one time. What *Tessier* called the "critical mass" measures about 1 cm^3. All portions of the graft must be within 5 mm of the blood supply, and two (but not three) of the dimensions of the graft may exceed 1 cm. Therefore, two or three stages of reconstruction are often necessary in cases of extreme bone defects.

The stability of the graft is essential for bone healing. Stabilization can be achieved by self-retention devices and/or osteosynthesis devices such as plates, screws and wires. Plates and screws are preferable to wires, because they provide easier and

stronger fixation. Macroplates are very useful to bridge a bone defect of the mandible. These materials are made of titanium or vitallium and can be left in place indefinitely. However, they are usually removed at the time of implant installation. When the implants are placed at the same time as the bone graft, one or two screws may first be used to temporarily fix the graft and are then replaced by implants (Fig. 3a and b).

(3) The coverage of the graft is provided by local flaps which are closed in one or, if possible, two layers. Incision of the periosteum is necessary for adequate mobilization of the flap. Excessive tension in the sutures will result in wound dehiscence after a few days. Again, any dead space between the graft and the flap must be avoided. Additional bone graft or vascularized soft tissues such as the buccal fat pad, temporalis or sternomastoid muscle flaps may be used to fill any empty space and protect the graft.

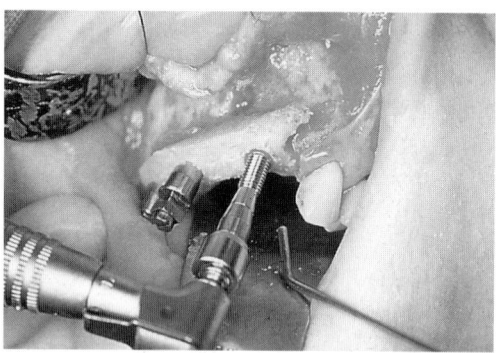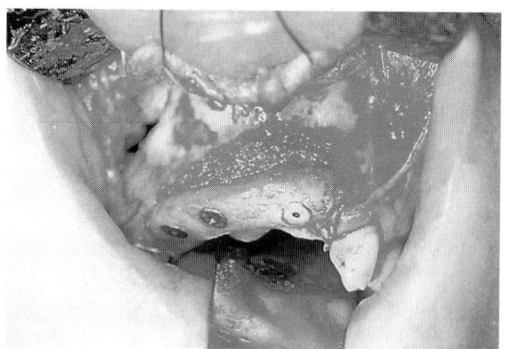

Fig. 3. (a) The implants are placed through the graft. (b) The depressed area above the graft is filled with cancellous bone to prevent a dead space after coverage of the graft. (Courtesy of Cahiers de Prothèse, № 71, Septembre 1990).

Methods of maxillofacial reconstruction

Patients with maxillofacial mutilations, whether congenital, or following trauma or resection of tumours, usually have associated bone and soft tissue defects.
Reconstruction with autogenous bone grafts and local or regional flaps is the only safe and predictable method in the long term. Bone substitutes may be helpful in some circumstances, but they carry an increased risk of infection, displacement and late extrusion. It is preferable not to use them, particularly when implant installation is planned in the reconstructed area.

Bone grafts

In facial surgery, bone grafts are usually taken from the chin, the ileum or the calvaria. The advantages and disadvantages of each type of bone are summarized in Table I.

Table I. Advantages and disadvantages of various types of bone grafts

	Nature	Volume	Pain	Scar	Hospital stay
Iliac	Cortical + Cancellous +++	+++	+	+	4–5 days
Cranium	Cortical +++ Cancellous +	+++	0	0	2–3 days
Chin	Cortical +++	+	0	0	1 day

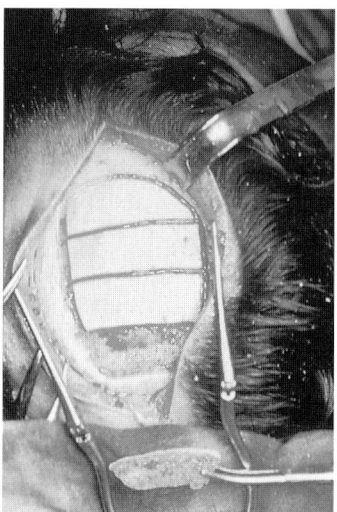 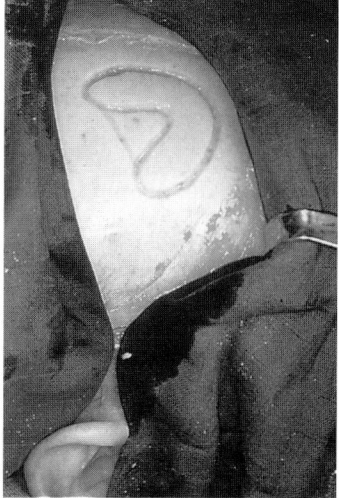 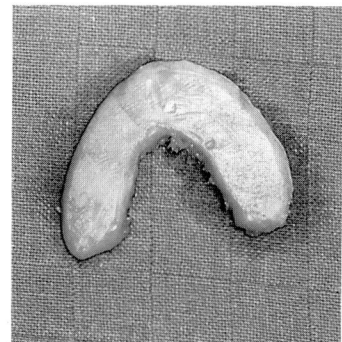

Fig. 4. (a) Harvesting cranial grafts in the right parietal region. (b) and (c) The calvaria can provide cortical, cancellous and cortico-cancellous grafts of various shapes. (Courtesy of Cahiers de Prothèse, Nº 71, Septembre 1990.)

The chin is a good source of bone. It is nearby and the procedure is absolutely painless. Of course, only a moderate amount of bone can be harvested, so that bone grafts from the chin are used exclusively to fill small defects.

The iliac graft is often still the material of choice for bone grafting. It is easily bent and contoured and can therefore be adapted to the most irregular recipient sites. It is necessary to take the crest itself, which is the dense part of the ilium, but the lateral lip of the crest must be left intact to prevent a contour deformity of the hip. The procedure is less painful when the muscular attachments are preserved.

The cranium is also a good bone graft source for facial skeletal surgery.[1] There is plenty of bone available, it is nearby, and can be taken without leaving a visible scar. The procedure is almost painless. Morphogenetically, it is the same sort of bone as most of the facial bones. The only drawback is that it is not particularly malleable compared to iliac bone or rib. The parietal-occipital area over the non-dominant hemisphere is the usual donor area, as the bone is thickest there.

The design of the graft may be rectangular or U-shaped, according to the anatomy of the recipient site (Fig. 4). The dense cranial bone provides excellent anchorage for oral implants.

Soft tissue flaps

Vestibular flaps[2], cervical flaps and temporalis muscle flaps are commonly used in the maxillo-mandibular area, but lie outside the scope of this book.

Microvascular osteomyocutaneous grafts

Free vascularized bone grafts from the iliac crest are indicated in the repair of large mandibular defects, particularly if the local conditions at the recipient site are poor, and there is a history of infection or radiotherapy. The possibility of simultaneous soft tissue transplantation is interesting when the defect involves a large cutaneous area[3].

New procedures and devices

New procedures include:

(1) Harvesting bone grafts from the calvaria. This donor site is particularly useful for the reconstruction of the jaws because of the extremely dense bone, which provides a strong anchorage for oral implants.

(2) The use of the temporalis muscle to fill large defects resulting from trauma or resection of tumours.

Cranial bone grafts and temporalis muscle flaps have been used extensively in craniofacial and maxillofacial surgery, since 1980[4, 5, 6].

New devices include:

(1) Osteosynthesis plates and screws, usually made of titanium and available in different sizes: micro, mini, maxi. They can be used to secure bone grafts and stabilize bone segments more strongly and rapidly than wires[7, 8].

(2) Osseointegrated implants have created a totally new range of possibilities for the functional rehabilitation of patients.

Conclusions

Before osseointegration was introduced, patients with severe mutilations of the maxillofacial region could benefit from reconstruction of bone and soft tissue, but attempts at prosthetic rehabilitation in these patients were frequently unsuccessful. With the application of osseointegration principles, the maxillofacial surgeon can achieve a much more satisfying result, both morphologically and functionally.

References

[1] Wolfe, S. A., Berkowitz, S. Plastic surgery of the facial skeleton. Boston: Little Brown and Co., 1989.

[2] Worthington, Ph. Hemimandibulectomy. In: Worthington, Ph., Brånemark, P.-I. (eds). Advanced osseointegration surgery: applications in the maxillofacial region. Ch. 22; pp. 259–266. Chicago: Quintessence Publ Co, 1992.

[3] Neukam, F. W., Hausamen, J. E. Microvascular bone grafting techniques in combination with osseointegrated fixtures. In: Worthington, Ph., Brånemark, P.-I. (eds). Ch. 24; pp. 276–292. Chicago: Quintessence Publ Co, 1992.

[4] Tessier, P. Present status and future prospects of cranio-facial surgery. Transactions of the Seventh International Congress of Plastic and Reconstructive Surgery. Rio de Janeiro, May 20–25, 1979.

[5] Tessier, P. Autogenous bone grafts taken from the calvarium for facial and cranial applications. Clin Plast Surg 1982; 9: 531–537.

[6] Tessier, P., Tulasne, J. F. Craniofacial surgery update. pp. 13–31. Year Book Medical Publishers, Inc., 1986.

[7] Yaremchuck, M. J., Gruss, J. S., Manson, P. N. Rigid fixation of the craniomaxillofacial skeleton. Boston: Butterworth-Heinemann, 1992.

[8] Tulasne, J. F., Tessier, P. Stability of skeletal fixation in congenital craniofacial surgery. In: Yaremchuck, M. J., Gruss, J. S., Manson, P. N. (eds). Rigid fixation of the craniomaxillofacial skeleton. pp. 507–511. Boston: Butterworth-Heinemann, 1992.

Chapter 12

Extra-oral applications of osseointegration

P.-I. Brånemark

Surgical procedures involving external maxillofacial defects which cannot be reconstructed using biological tissue, require prosthetic substitution. The optimal function of anatomically correct synthetic components requires reliable mechanical retention of the prosthesis.

Over the years, procedures have been developed in which titanium retention elements have been installed in the bone tissue close to the defect, thus providing anchorage for the prosthesis through mechanical or magnetic retention. In some cases, bone grafting procedures and special skin trimming procedures have to be used, in order to provide adequate mechanical stability and to ensure a reaction-free connection where the abutment pierces the skin[1, 2] (Figs 1 and 2).

A wide variety of defects exist; ranging from congenital, surgical or traumatic absence or loss of either ear, nose or orbit, to major facial defects, sometimes in combination with oral abnormalities (Figs 3–6).

Major intra-oral defects such as total or partial maxillectomy can be reconstructed using a combination of autologous bone grafts and specially designed anchorage elements and prostheses (Fig. 7).

Osseointegration has also been used to provide retention for bone-conduction hearing aids. Conventional arrangement using a spring-loaded attachment across the head often causes inconvenience and pain because of compression of the soft tissue. The skin also reduces the quality of the signal provided by the hearing aid, when entering the skull bone. An osseointegrated titanium implant in the mastoid bone behind the ear has proved to be a realistic alternative, giving better retention and improving the quality of transfer of the acoustic signal[3] (Fig. 8).

Based on long-term clinical experience of osseointegration in the oral and craniomaxillofacial region, titanium implants have also been used for the retention of joint prostheses, particularly in finger and ankle joints, and for amputation prostheses in the limbs (Figs 9–12).

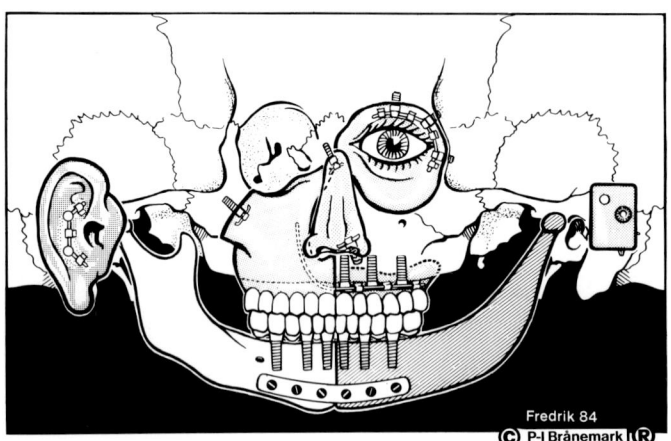

Fig. 1a

Fredrik 84
© P-I Brånemark ®

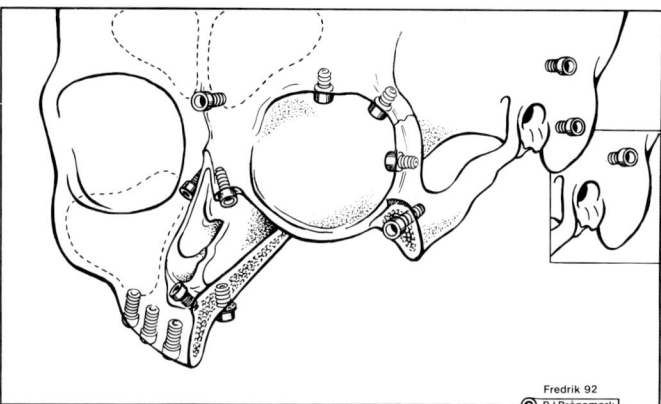

Fig. 1b

Fredrik 92
© P-I Brånemark

Fig. 1. (a) Diagram summarizing the rehabilitation modalities in the oral and maxillofacial region with the aid of tissue-integrated prostheses; (b) topographical location of implants for the retention of bone-anchored hearing aids and prostheses in maxillofacial reconstruction: maxilla, nose, orbit, midface, ear[4].

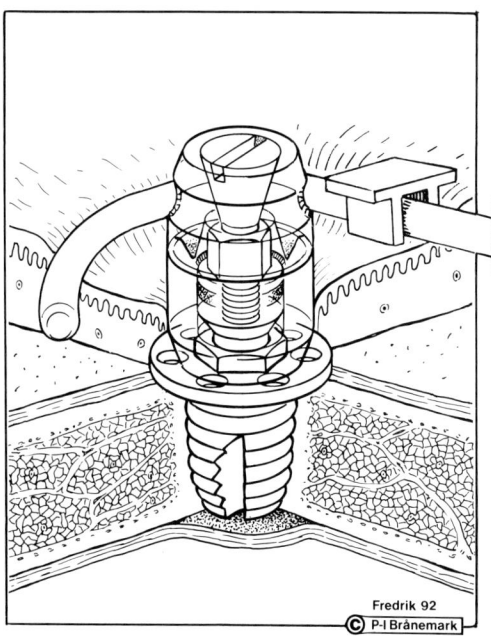

Fredrik 92
© P-I Brånemark

Fig. 2. Schematic summary of specially designed anchorage elements for retention in the skull bone. The implant has a flange to improve anchorage and minimize the risk of intrusion in case of external injury. The components are firmly connected using screw attachments and a removable metal bar.

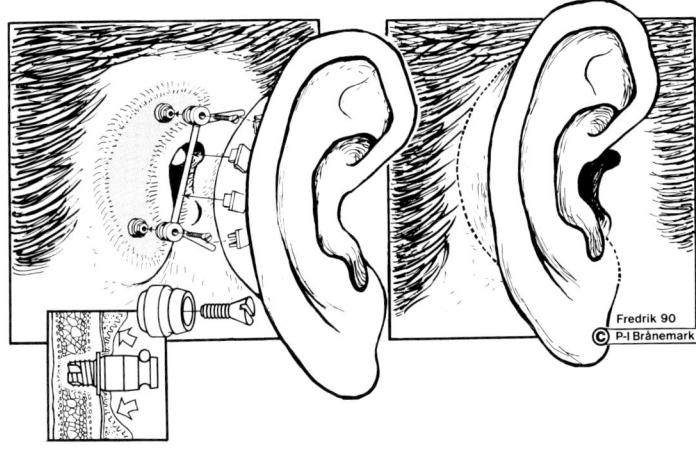

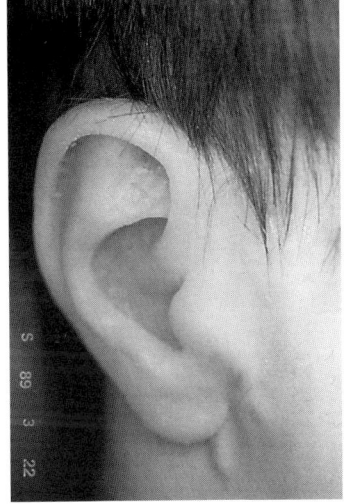
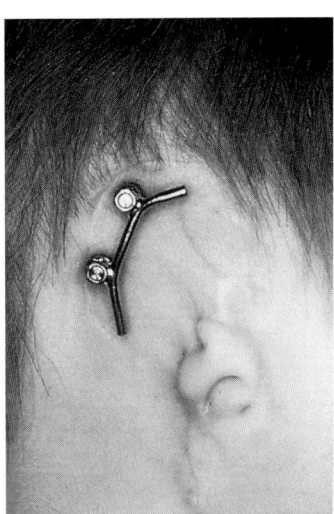

Fig. 3. Example of a bone-anchored ear prosthesis and clinical example of an artificial ear anchored via a bar to two integrated implants behind the ear.

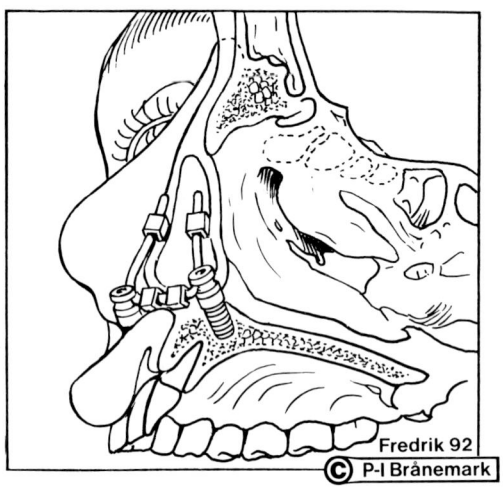

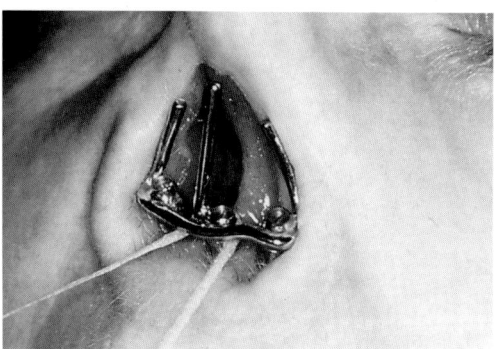

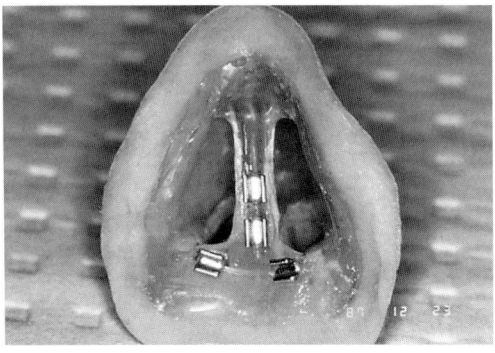

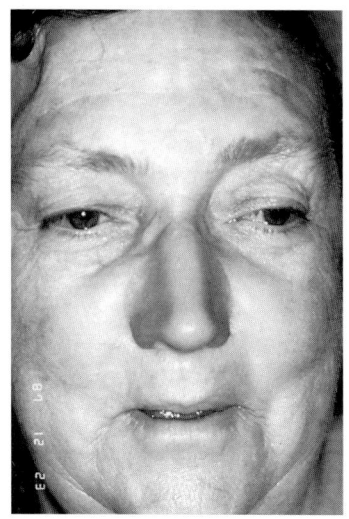

Fig. 4. Positioning of implants connected via a metal bar to carry a nose prosthesis using clip retention.

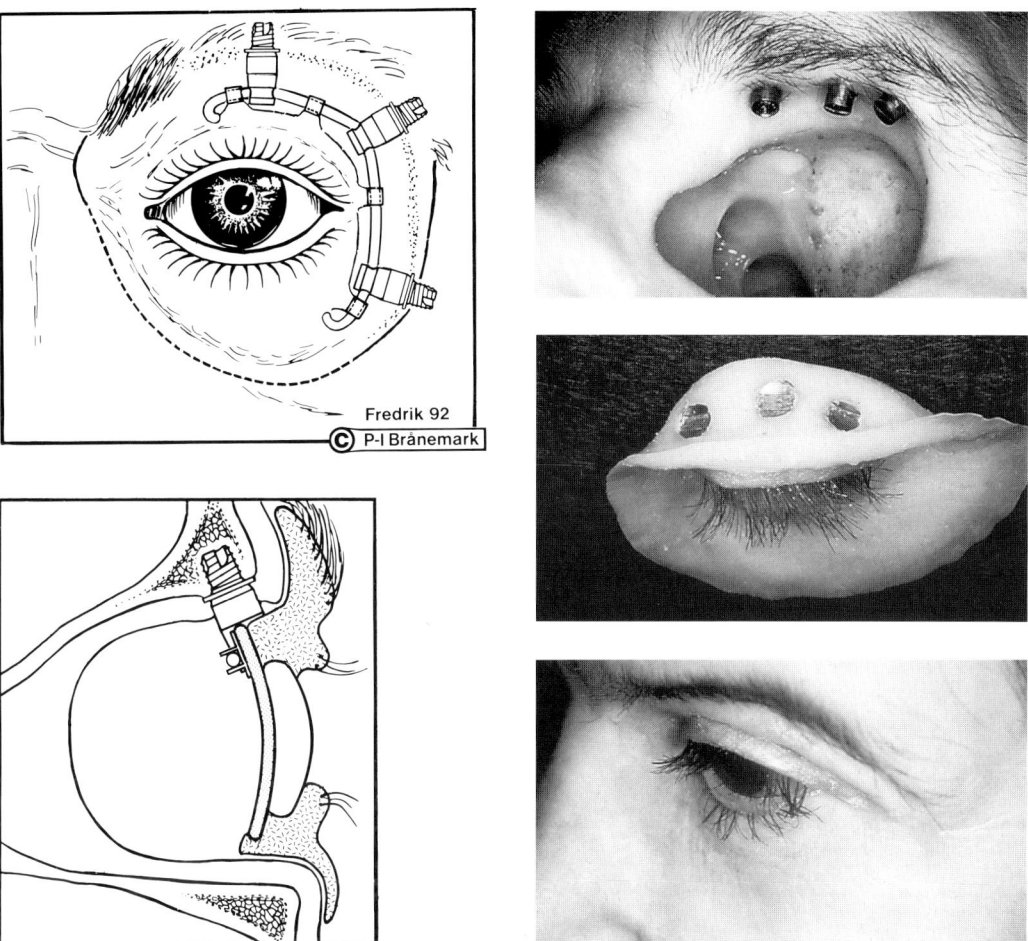

Fig. 5. Prosthetic replacement of the orbit. It is important to position the implants in such a way that the outer contour of the prosthesis is not affected by protruding mechanical elements.

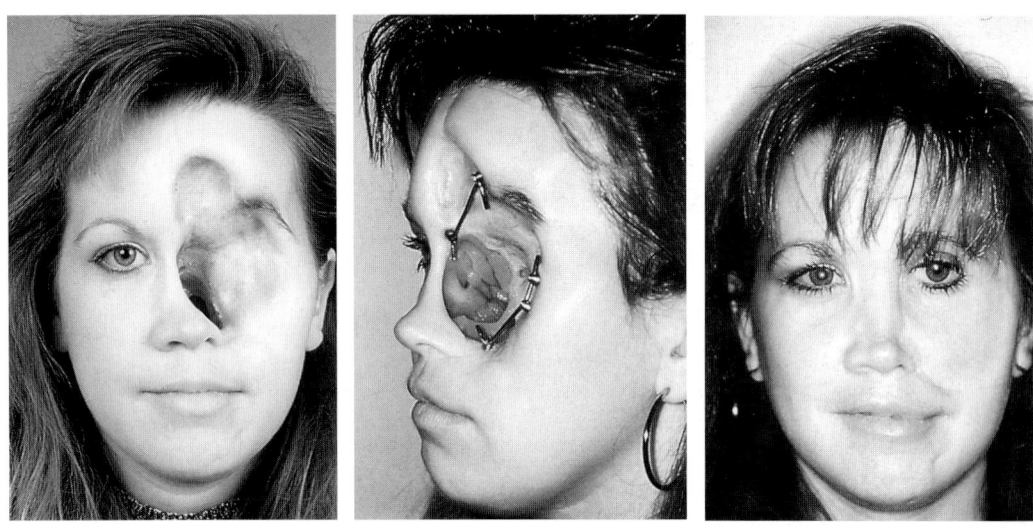

Fig. 6. A major facial defect following tumour resection can be fitted with a prosthesis retained via a few endosseous fixtures. It is imperative that external maxillofacial prostheses mimic the normal situation in anatomy and texture.

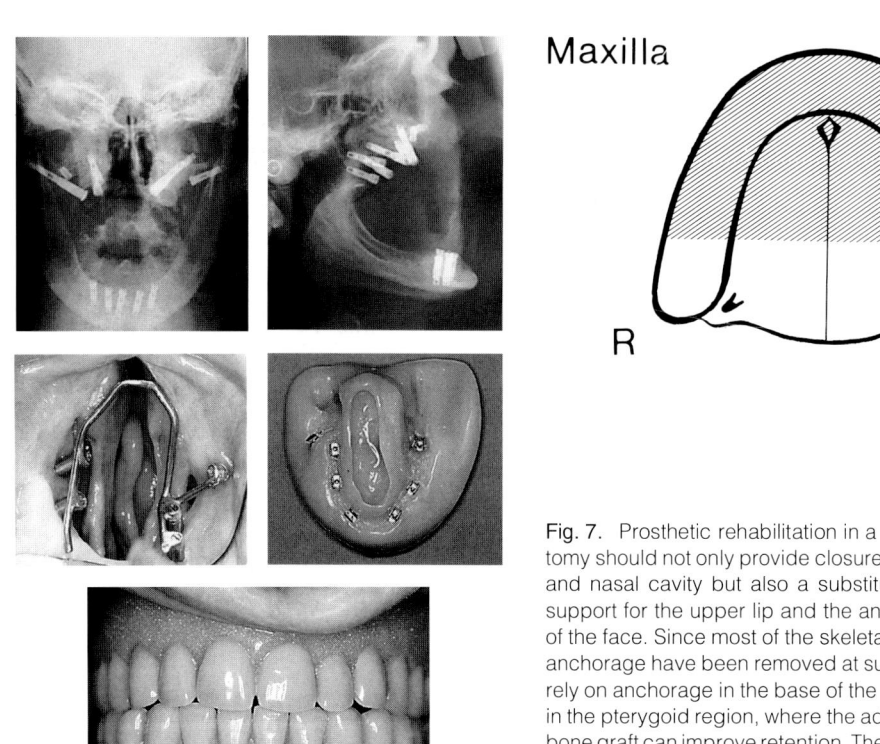

Maxilla

R   L

Fig. 7. Prosthetic rehabilitation in a case of maxillectomy should not only provide closure between the oral and nasal cavity but also a substitute for teeth and support for the upper lip and the anterior soft tissues of the face. Since most of the skeletal components for anchorage have been removed at surgery, one has to rely on anchorage in the base of the zygoma and also in the pterygoid region, where the addition of an onlay bone graft can improve retention. The prostheses have to be carefully and continuously adjusted to fit the defect and to prevent leakage between the oral and nasal cavity.

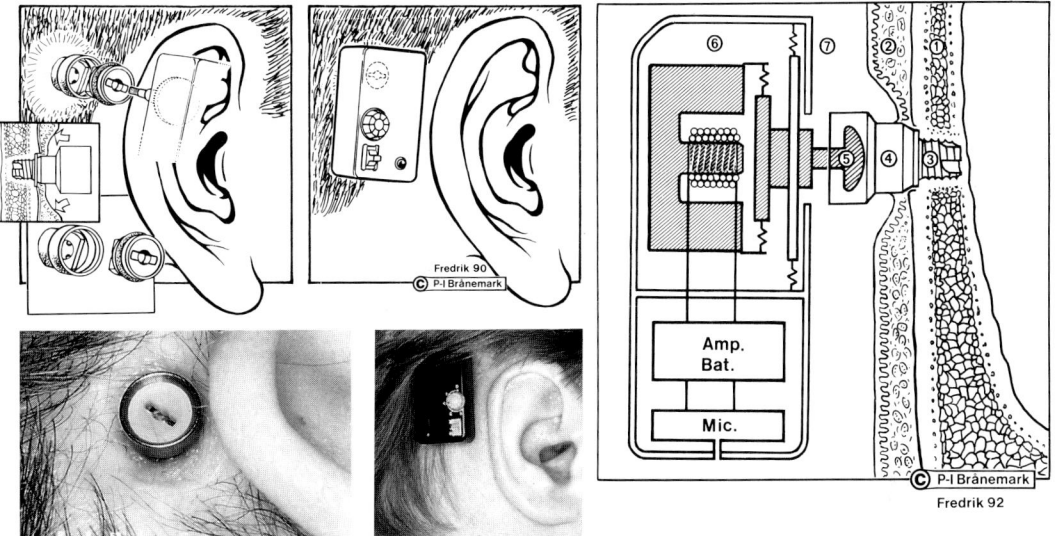

Fig. 8. A bone-anchored hearing aid. A single implant, provided with a special abutment for connection of hearing aid, transfers the acoustic signal to the inner ear. Rejection-free skin penetration often requires careful trimming of the skin to provide immobile soft tissue.

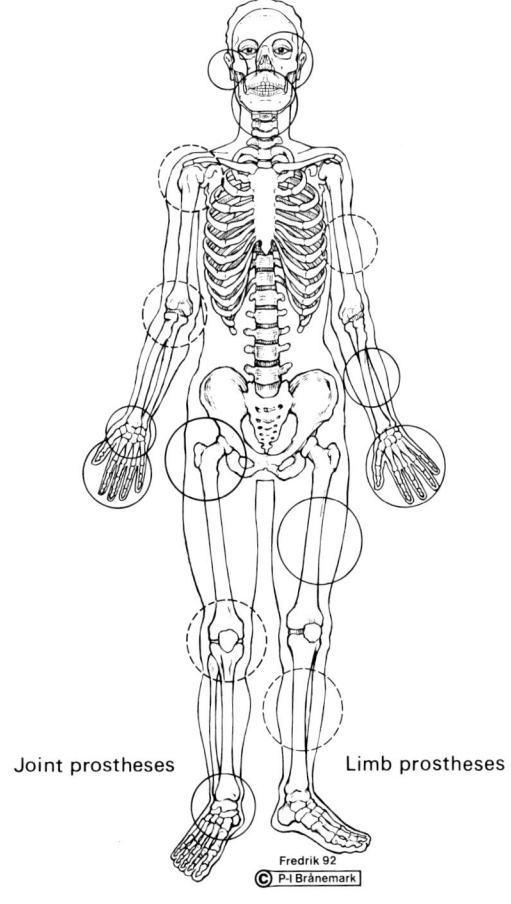

Fig. 9. Osseointegrated prostheses have been used outside the cranio-maxillofacial region, in hand surgery and orthopaedics.

199

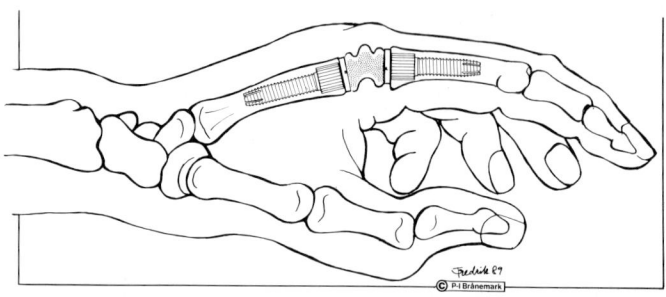

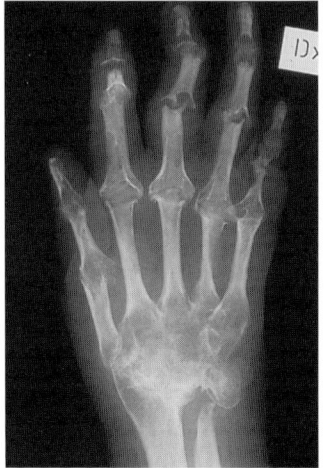

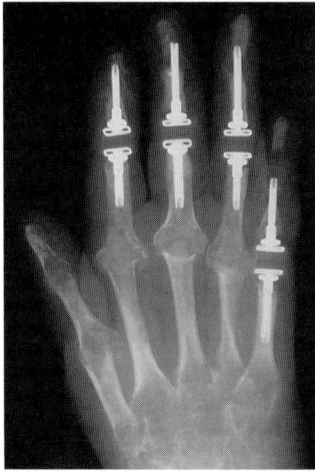

Fig. 10. Diseased or damaged finger joints can be replaced by a synthetic joint mechanism that is anchored to the neighbouring digital ones via implants in the medullary cavity. Stable anchorage results in controlled function of the joint without continuing resorption of the bone. Because of the mechanical design, the joint mechanism can be replaced in case of wear or mechanical failure.

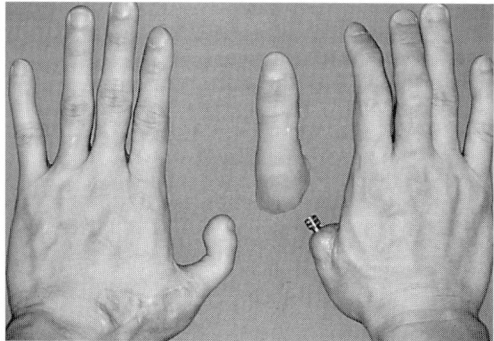

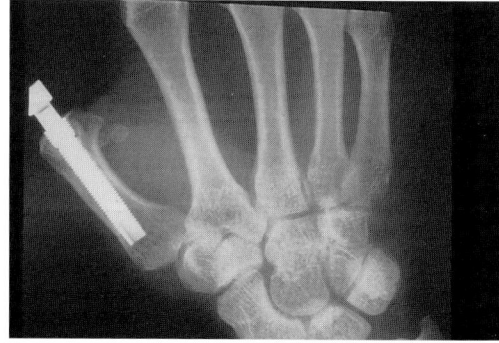

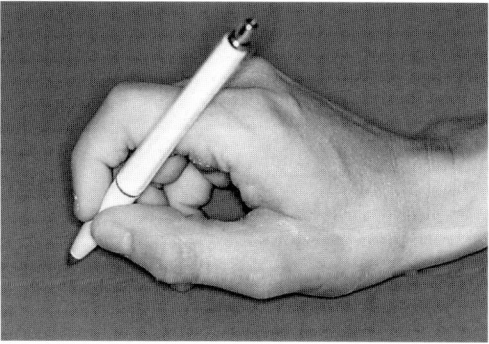

Fig. 11. Bilateral thumb amputation with transplantation of the second toe from both feet using microvascular anastomoses. Failure occurred in the right hand. A titanium implant was anchored in the remaining skeletal bone of the base of the thumb. A prosthesis directly connected to the implant provides the patient with good overall function of the hand; with a stable prosthesis and even some proprioceptive function.

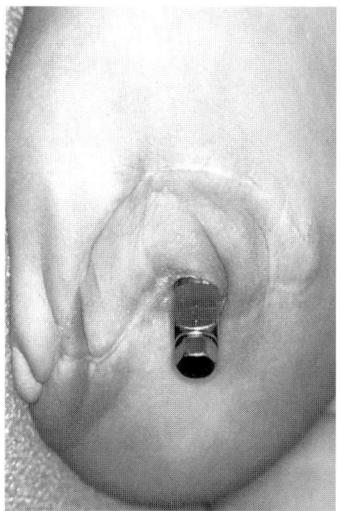 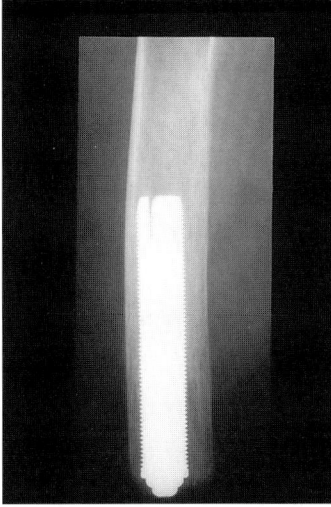 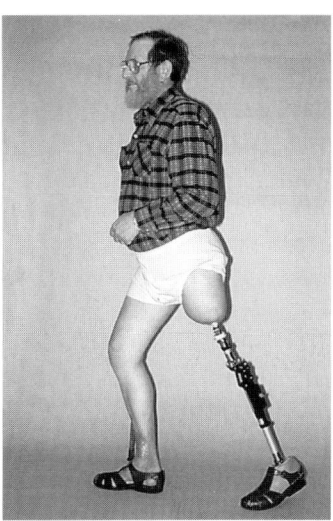

Fig. 12. A femur amputee who experienced difficulties with a conventional limb prosthesis was provided with an anchorage implant in what remained of the femur. Using special mechanical connectors, a prosthesis was directly connected to the bone. This procedure not only resulted in mechanical stability without adverse tissue reactions, but also provided the patient with a certain amount of sensory perception via the osseointegrated reconstruction.

References

[1] Tjellström, A. Osseointegrated systems and their applications in the head and neck. Adv Otolaryngol Head Neck Surg 1989; 3: 39–70.

[2] Worthington, P., Brånemark, P.-I. (eds). Advanced osseointegration surgery: applications in the maxillo-facial region. Chicago: Quintessence Publ Co, Inc, 1992.

[3] Håkansson, B., Lidén, G., Tjellström, A., Ringdahl, A., Jacobsson, M., Carlsson, P., Erlandson, B.-E. 10 years of experience with the Swedish bone anchored hearing system. Ann Otolaryngol 1990; 99: 10 Part II (suppl. 151).

[4] Brånemark, P.-I., Zarb, G. and Albrektsson, T. (eds). Tissue-integrated prostheses. Osseointegration in clinical dentistry. Chicago: Quintessence Publ. Co, 1985.

Index

A

B

C